# Managing Your Substance Use Disorder

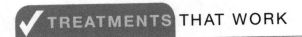 TREATMENTS THAT WORK

# Managing Your Substance Use Disorder

## Third Edition

CLIENT WORKBOOK

DENNIS C. DALEY
ANTOINE DOUAIHY

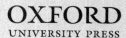

OXFORD
UNIVERSITY PRESS

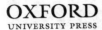

OXFORD
UNIVERSITY PRESS

Oxford University Press is a department of the University of Oxford. It furthers
the University's objective of excellence in research, scholarship, and education
by publishing worldwide. Oxford is a registered trade mark of Oxford University
Press in the UK and certain other countries.

Published in the United States of America by Oxford University Press
198 Madison Avenue, New York, NY 10016, United States of America.

CIP data is on file at the Library of Congress
ISBN 978–0–19–092667–0

9 8 7 6 5 4 3 2 1

Printed by Marquis, Canada

# About ✓TREATMENTS THAT WORK

One of the most difficult problems confronting patients with various disorders and diseases is finding the best help available. Everyone is aware of friends or family who have sought treatment from a seemingly reputable practitioner, only to find out later from another doctor that the original diagnosis was wrong or the treatments recommended were inappropriate or perhaps even harmful. Most patients, or family members, address this problem by reading everything they can about their symptoms, seeking out information on the Internet, or aggressively "asking around" to tap knowledge from friends and acquaintances. Governments and healthcare policy-makers are also aware that people in need don't always get the best treatments, something they refer to as "variability in healthcare practices."

Now healthcare systems around the world are attempting to correct this variability by introducing "evidence-based practice." This simply means that it is in everyone's interest that patients get the most up-to-date and effective care for a particular problem. Healthcare policy-makers have also recognized that it is very useful to give consumers of healthcare as much information as possible, so that they can make intelligent decisions in a collaborative effort to improve health and mental health. This series, *Treatments That Work,* is designed to accomplish just that. Only the latest and most effective interventions for particular problems are described in user-friendly language. To be included in this series, each treatment program must pass the highest standards of evidence available, as determined by a scientific advisory board. Thus, when individuals suffering from these problems or their family members seek out an expert clinician who is familiar with these interventions and decides that they are appropriate, they will have confidence that they are receiving the best care available. Of course, only your healthcare professional can decide on the right mix of treatments for you.

The ravages of substance use disorder have been documented time and again, and the lives ruined are too numerous to count. But new treatment programs have appeared in the last decade that have been proven to be effective in relieving the burden of substance use disorder for a large number of individuals. The program described in this Workbook presents the latest version of one of the most advanced treatment programs yet developed for substance use disorder. This program recognizes that these problems have both biological and psychological causes, and that no single program will work the same for everyone. Therefore it is meant to be flexibly adapted to wherever the individual is on the long road to recovery, from just getting started through preventing relapse. Incorporating the wisdom of programs that have come before such as 12-step programs, cognitive-behavioral programs, and relapse prevention approaches, this treatment benefits from decades of development and scientific evaluation and has been used to the benefit of thousands of individuals with these problems. In this program you will learn skills to cope effectively with cues and triggers that lead to use and abuse of drugs and alcohol and hopefully master the emotional roller coaster that accompanies this condition. This includes altering patterns of beliefs, dealing with interpersonal conflicts that often lead to use and addiction, and building healthy social support systems. This program is most effectively applied by working in collaboration with your clinician.

David H. Barlow, Editor-in-Chief,
Treatments *ThatWork*
Boston, MA

## Accessing Treatments *ThatWork* Forms and Worksheets Online

All forms and worksheets from books in the Treatments *ThatWork* (TTW) series are made available digitally shortly following print publication. You may download, print, save, and digitally complete them as PDFs. To access the forms and worksheets, please visit http://www.oup.com/us/ttw.

# Contents

# Managing Your Substance Use Disorder

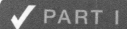

# PART I

# Overview of Substance Use Problems and Assessment

## CHAPTER 1

Introduction and Plan for This Workbook

## Goals

- To become aware of current trends in substance use, misuse, and substance use disorders
- To learn the multiple factors contributing to a substance problem
- To identify the different paths and benefits to recovery
- To understand the benefits of using this workbook in therapy or counseling
- To learn the importance of keeping records and completing recovery worksheets

## Introduction and Overview

This recovery workbook provides you with practical information and skills to help you understand and change your problem with alcohol, tobacco, or other drugs such as marijuana, cocaine or methamphetamine, heroin or fentanyl, or nonprescribed addictive medications. It is designed to be used in therapy or counseling and will help you focus on specific issues involved in stopping substance use and in changing behaviors that keep your substance use problem active. The information presented in this workbook is derived from research, clinical and recovery literature, and our many years of experience working with clients who have alcohol, tobacco, and other drug problems. It discusses the most effective and helpful recovery issues and change strategies from studies of cognitive-behavioral treatment, coping skills training, 12-step counseling, and relapse prevention. These treatment approaches focus on the importance of changing beliefs, thinking, relationships, and behaviors and learning "skills" to help you stay sober and change your life. Such changes not only help you initiate and sustain recovery but also improve the quality of your life.

Your recovery change plan should be tailored to your needs and problems. No single recovery program is for everyone. There are many paths to recovery. The ideas in this workbook will help you work with a therapist or counselor to develop your personal plan for recovery based on the severity of your substance use problem, your motivation to change, and your willingness to work diligently in improving yourself.

In this workbook, we provide you with information about substance use problems, recovery, relapse, professional treatments available, and mutual support programs. When we talk about "substance use problems," we are referring to problems with alcohol, tobacco, or any other type of drug. Problems may show in binge drinking, drug misuse (using illicit drugs, using other people's prescription drugs with addiction potential, mixing drugs or drugs and alcohol in ways that are risky) or a substance use disorder (SUD). Although there are differences among the various substance use problems, there are also many similarities. Therefore, the recovery strategies discussed throughout this workbook can be adapted to any type of substance-related problem. The goals of this workbook are to help you reach maximum treatment benefit by motivating you to develop and implement a personal change plan and to provide you with practical strategies and skills to cope with the most common problems and challenges encountered when substance use is stopped.

This workbook includes the following topics:

- Recognizing your substance use problem and the consequences of it
- Choosing the right treatment setting
- Managing your cravings to use alcohol, tobacco, or other drugs
- Controlling thoughts of using alcohol or drugs and managing obsessions to use
- Dealing with upsetting emotions (anger, boredom, depression, and so on)
- Refusing offers to use substances and not giving in to social pressures
- Dealing with family and interpersonal conflicts
- Building a recovery support system to establish a "we" program
- Identifying and managing relapse warning signs to catch them early

- Identifying and managing your unique high-risk relapse factors
- Taking action quickly if you use again to limit the severity and damage of a relapse
- Living a balanced life so you gain pleasure and satisfaction from nonchemical activities
- Measuring your progress
- Managing a coexisting psychiatric disorder or behavioral addiction (e.g., gambling, internet, sex, or spending)

## Extent of Substance Use Problems

A substance use problem exists when you experience any type of difficulty related to using alcohol, tobacco, or other drugs, including illicit street drugs or prescribed drugs such as painkillers (opioids), tranquilizers (used for anxiety), sedatives (used for sleep), or stimulants (used for attention deficit disorder or weight control). The difficulty can be in any area of your life: medical or physical, psychological, family, interpersonal, social, academic, occupational, legal, financial, or spiritual.

### Extent of Substance Use and Substance Use Disorders

Surveys conducted each year by the Substance Abuse and Mental Health Services Administration (SAMHSA) and other studies or reports found the following:

- In 2015, about 44.5% or 119 million adults in the United States used one of four medications with addiction potential mentioned earlier; the majority got these drugs from a family member or friend or purchased these from a drug dealer.
- After alcohol and tobacco, the most common drugs misused are marijuana, pain pills, cocaine or methamphetamine, stimulant medications, heroin or fentanyl, or prescribed sedatives. Rates of use of all of these drugs—except pain medications—are rising.
- While only about 11% of those ages 12 or older used illicit drugs, 25% of individuals ages 18–25 used illicit drugs, making this a group at risk for substance use disorders.
- There are more than 136 million current alcohol users in the United States. More than 65 million had an episode of "binge" drinking (4 or more during a drinking occasion for a woman or a man over age 65; 5 or more drinks for a man under age 65); more than 16 million

had multiple binge episodes; and 20% of young people between 12 and 20 drink alcohol.

- More than 20 million people had a substance use disorder (SUD) in the past year, which is about 7.5% of the population ages 12 and above. The next chapter will provide specific symptoms of a SUD, which refers to a "pattern of substance use" that causes problems and distress and is characterized by up to 11 symptoms.
- Rates of alcohol use disorder are the highest, with more than 15 million having this problem compared to 7.4 million who had a drug use disorder.
- Only 10.6% of those with a SUD receive treatment in specialty addiction programs. However, in recent years, due to the opioid epidemic, many individuals with opioid addiction are receiving medication-assisted treatment from medical practitioners in hospitals or primary care clinics.
- Unfortunately, only a few percent of individuals with a SUD believe they need help, which means that families, employers, friends, or the legal system must influence them to get help. Since you are in treatment, you have the opportunity to learn strategies to manage your substance problems *and* improve your life significantly.
- Rates of death from drug overdose (OD) continue to rise each year, with more than 64,000 dying from ODs in 2017, mainly from illicit opioids like heroin or fentanyl, often mixed with other potent drugs like tranquilizers.

SUDs can cause or worsen problems in any area of life. These will be reviewed in Chapter 3 of this workbook to help you understand the effects of your substance problem on different areas of your life.

## Overcoming a Substance Problem: Paths to Recovery

The good news is that there are many paths to recovery from a substance problem and these benefit millions of people. These paths include professional treatment (counseling, therapy, a "program," medications, or a combination of these), mutual support programs, peer-assisted recovery (peer navigators, coaches, specialists), and self-recovery. The more severe the substance problem, the more likely professional treatment is needed in addition to other strategies.

A recent study published by the Harvard Research Recovery Institute found that more than 22 million adults in the United States who once had a SUD no longer have one. Their paths to recovery include the following:

- 45% used mutual support programs
- 28% used professional treatment
- 9% used medications (e.g., for alcohol, opioid, or tobacco use disorders)

Many people use a combination of these strategies. What is impressive is that 29% have more than 15 years of recovery, and an additional 35% have between 5 and 15 years of recovery. Many studies of treatment and surveys of individuals in recovery in the United States, Australia, Canada, and the United Kingdom show that involvement in treatment and/or recovery services often leads to dramatic improvements in all areas of life, such as

- Improved physical and dental health and higher engagement in healthy behaviors
- Improved mental health and higher engagement in mental health treatment
- Improved family relationships (more shared activities, much less violence)
- Improvement in work or school (steady employment, finishing school, starting a business)
- Improved financial condition (pay bills, debts, or taxes; save for the future)
- Fewer illegal activities, arrests, driving under the influence of alcohol or drug episodes, less use of medical emergency room visits, and increased rates of medical insurance

## Causes of Substance Use Problems

There is no single cause of all alcohol or drug problems. These problems are caused by a number of different biological, psychological, and social or environmental factors that vary from one person to the next.

### Biological Causes

Alcohol problems run in families, so it is thought that some individuals have a genetic predisposition to develop an alcohol problem. Keep in mind that no one specific "alcohol" or "drug dependence" gene has yet been identified. However, it is likely that there are differences in brain chemistry and metabolism that increase the likelihood of developing an addiction to alcohol or other substances (*addiction* is usually referred to as a more severe substance use disorder). Scientists believe that these addictive substances work on the *mesolimbic dopamine* pathway or "reward" pathway of the brain. This is the part of the brain that makes food, sex, and social activities pleasurable. As addiction progresses, the brain is "hijacked" by substances. The result is that the person with addiction relies more on substances and less on natural rewards to feel good. Even though substance use causes many problems, it is then "reinforced" when the person ingests alcohol or drugs. Some people with an addictive disorder also develop a tolerance for alcohol or other drugs, requiring an increasing amount of alcohol or drugs to obtain the desired effect. Their bodies seem to "need" or "want" substances, unlike people who do not develop an addiction or dependence on substances. Also, during active addiction, "memories" can trigger intense cravings for alcohol or drugs.

## Psychological Causes

Substances are often used to reduce anxiety or tension, to relax, to cope with other unpleasant feelings, or to escape. For some people, this eventually contributes to a SUD as they get more accustomed to using alcohol, tobacco, or other drugs to feel normal. Others have certain personality traits that make them more prone to using and subsequently misusing substances. Some have a psychiatric disorder, which can increase their vulnerability to developing a substance-related disorder.

## Social or Environmental Causes

The family and social environments in which we live influence most behaviors, including substance use behavior. A person's decision to use or not to use substances is affected by access to substances, pressure from peers to use, reinforcement from peers for using, observance of role models (e.g., parents) using or misusing substances, and standards or values learned from the community or broader culture.

## Multiple Causes

Most likely it is not one but a combination of factors that caused you to develop a substance use problem. In cases of more severe SUDs (e.g., addiction), the factors that contributed to your initial use may be different from those that cause you to continue using. For some people, physical factors may be the strongest, whereas for others psychological or social factors may be the strongest. Identifying the factors that contribute to your substance use problem can contribute to your recovery.

## Benefits of This Workbook

This workbook offers many benefits, especially when used with professional therapy or counseling:

- First, it will help you become more educated about substance use problems and recovery. Understanding the recovery process, for example, makes it easier to cope with the ups and downs you are likely to experience.
- Second, this workbook will help you look at your particular problem with alcohol, tobacco, or other drugs and identify how it has affected your life and the lives of people close to you.
- Third, it will help you learn specific skills to manage the challenges and "nuts and bolts" problems encountered in recovery.
- Finally, it will help you reduce the risk of a future lapse and relapse.

As a result of working a recovery program, you can experience benefits in your physical, emotional, or spiritual health; family and social relationships; ability to work or go to school; and legal and financial conditions. There are many potential short-term and long-term benefits of recovery.

### Tips on Using This Workbook in Your Treatment

This interactive recovery workbook was written to be used in conjunction with therapy or counseling. Ask your therapist or counselor for help in choosing which topics to work on and in what sequence. The sequence you choose should be based on your unique problems with substance use and where you are in the recovery process. If you have any questions about the meaning of the information presented, how it relates to your situation, or how to use it to aid your recovery, ask your therapist. If you try to implement some of the change strategies recommended and find they aren't working for you, work with your therapist to figure out why these ideas aren't helpful or if you need to find other strategies. Even if you don't agree with what you read in this workbook, you will find it helpful to discuss your reactions and ideas with your therapist.

This workbook can be used whether you are in individual or group therapy, or both. An open, honest, realistic, and disciplined approach to recovery in which you face your issues rather than avoid them will help you make the most progress.

Abstinence from the use of substances is usually the most appropriate goal of treatment, especially if you have a more severe SUD or addiction. However, some people initially benefit from a harm-reduction approach before they agree on abstinence. Harm reduction refers to a reduction in the amount and frequency of substance use so there is a reduction in the negative consequences such as medical, family, work, or legal problems. However, there is always the risk that serious consequences or even death could result if you do not stop completely.

## The Importance of Records and Completing Recovery Worksheets

Throughout this recovery workbook, you will be asked to complete several records and worksheets related to each area of recovery. These assignments have several purposes:

1. To help you personalize the information presented so that you relate it to your unique situation.
2. To help you become aware of the many aspects of recovery and of the relationships among thoughts, feelings, and behaviors. We emphasize biological, psychological, social, and spiritual aspects of recovery.
3. To help you identify internal and external triggers of substance use and develop strategies to manage them.
4. To provide you with a reminder that you need to take an active role in reducing or stopping alcohol and drug use and learn to cope positively with the problems experienced in recovery.
5. To help you carry out the proposed recovery change techniques and practice them in your daily life.
6. To help you document problems as well as successes with specific changes. Keeping track of your progress over time allows you to see the "big picture" and put setbacks into perspective. This also provides you with "accountability" so that you are reminded that it is up to you to continue to work at positive changes.

7. To help you approach your treatment in a systematic and structured way. This allows you to take maximum advantage of your therapy sessions because you are always working on important recovery issues between treatment sessions.

You may photocopy worksheets and records from the workbook or download additional copies from the Treatments *ThatWork*™ Web site at www. oup.com/us/ttw.

This interactive recovery workbook can be used as your personal notebook to keep track of important issues in your quest to manage your substance use problem. You can revisit sections of this workbook as many times as you need to help yourself develop and modify your change plan. When you are finished with professional treatment, this workbook can serve as a reminder for you. After a period of time, you can go back, review, and add to it as you learn new ways to handle the problems and demands of recovery. We applaud you for your interest in learning strategies to manage your substance use problem and improve the quality of your life.

## CHAPTER 2

# Recognizing Your Substance Use Problem

## Goals

- To understand the different categories and symptoms of substance use disorders
- To rate the overall severity of your substance use problem

## Continuum of Substance Use Problems

The American Psychiatric Association classifies substance-related disorders into several categories. These include intoxication, withdrawal, substance use disorder (SUD), and substance-induced disorder.

### Intoxication and Withdrawal

*Intoxication* refers to being "drunk," "stoned," "loaded," or "under the influence" of alcohol or other drugs. It involves physiological signs such as slurred speech and/or incoordination with alcohol or other sedatives or hypnotics; elevated blood pressure with cocaine or other stimulants; or drowsiness or slurred speech with opioids. Intoxication also involves psychological or behavioral changes such as aggressiveness, irritability, impaired attention, or disturbance of mood. Intoxication affects judgment and can contribute to serious behaviors such as violence toward others, accidents, or suicide attempts.

*Withdrawal* symptoms are caused by stopping or reducing the intake of substances that produce physical dependence (e.g., alcohol, heroin).

Specific withdrawal symptoms are discussed in Chapter 15 (which also addresses medications used in the treatment of substance use problems).

### Symptoms of Substance Use Disorder

If your pattern of substance use leads to significant impairment in your life or to personal distress, and you meet two or more of the symptoms listed in Worksheet 2.1: Substance Use Disorder Criteria, at the end of this chapter, you have a "substance use disorder." If you have 2–3 symptoms, your disorder is considered mild; with 4–5 symptoms, it is considered moderate; and with 6 or more symptoms, it is considered severe. As you read these criteria, note whether or not you have experienced each of them by placing a check mark in the appropriate box.

Worksheet 2.2: Self-Rating Scale, at the end of this chapter, can help you rate the overall severity of your substance use problem. Also, the effects of substance use can vary from one person to the next, from mild to life-threatening.

### Substance-Induced Disorders

The effects of alcohol and other drugs on the central nervous system can cause substance-induced mood, anxiety, and psychotic disorders or magnify personality disorders. What this means is that symptoms that look like a psychiatric illness develop but then clear up with continued abstinence from alcohol or other drugs. Therefore several weeks or longer is often needed to determine if a depression or anxiety syndrome is an independent psychiatric disorder or is caused by the chronic use of substances. For example, Matt felt extremely depressed and suicidal following several weeks of using cocaine daily. However, within a week of stopping cocaine and entering a recovery program, his mood improved significantly. On the other hand, Shannon stopped drinking alcohol and using tranquilizers, and the longer she was sober, the more anxious and depressed she became. Shannon was clearly suffering from psychiatric problems in addition to her dependence on substances. Her use of alcohol and tranquilizers was her way of coping with her symptoms through "self-medicating."

### Homework

✎ Complete Worksheet 2.2: Self-Rating Scale.

## Worksheet 2.1
## Substance Use Disorder Criteria

### Criterion 1: Loss of Control                    ☐ Yes    ☐ No

You use a greater quantity of alcohol or drugs than you intended or for longer periods of time than you intended. Examples: Ron bought an ounce of marijuana and planned to use it over a period of several weeks but ended up smoking it all in a few days. Lisa constantly tells herself she's going to have only a few drinks at parties each weekend, but she always gets drunk.

### Criterion 2: Can't Cut Down or Control Use        ☐ Yes    ☐ No

You have a persistent desire or unsuccessful efforts to cut down or control your alcohol or drug use. You may quit, only to go back to using again. Examples: Dennis has quit smoking at least 10 times in the past few years for periods from several days to 3 months, but he always goes back to smoking. Liz buys a rock of crack cocaine when she gets her check with the intention of not smoking more than that. However, she ends up purchasing more crack and more often than not uses her entire check to buy the drug, smoking continuously until she runs out of drugs and money.

### Criterion 3: Preoccupation or Compulsion           ☐ Yes    ☐ No

You spend a great deal of time on activities necessary to obtain the substance, use the substance, or recover from its effects. Examples: Sandy, a nurse, spends a considerable amount of time figuring out ways to steal narcotic drugs at work. Stephen plans his work day so that he's able to use cocaine. Also, his weekends are almost entirely dedicated to getting high on drugs.

### Criterion 4: Craving                               ☐ Yes    ☐ No

You have strong desires or urges to drink alcohol or use drugs. Examples: Even though Jack has not had a drink in several weeks, he has strong cravings nearly every day. Jessica stopped using pain pills but still feels strong desires to get some even though she knows this will worsen her addiction.

### Criterion 5: Fail to Fulfill Major Obligations     ☐ Yes    ☐ No

You do not fulfill your obligations at work, home, or school. Examples: Chris's cannabis problem led to poor grades and dropping out of college. Megan often depends on her teenage daughter to babysit Megan's 8-year-old while she goes out drinking with friends, often staying out late.

**Criterion 6: Continued Use Despite Problems**　　　　☐ **Yes**　　☐ **No**

You have recurrent social or relationship problems that are caused by or worsened by substance use. Examples: During episodes of drunkenness, Dan instigates fights in bars or at parties. He has a reputation of being unpredictable when he drinks too much. Rebecca left her husband because he refused to get help for his addiction. She felt like he was ruining their marriage because he was often gone and she felt she could not trust him.

**Criterion 7: Psychosocial Impairment**　　　　☐Yes　　☐ **No**

You give up or lose important social, occupational, or recreational activities because of substance use. Examples: Melissa has lost two jobs due to absenteeism caused by alcohol use. She has also quit swimming and playing tennis. Leonard was kicked off the football team because he tested positive for drugs on three different occasions. As a result, he also lost his scholarship and dropped out of college.

**Criterion 8: Use in Hazardous Situations**　　　　☐ **Yes**　　☐ **No**

You use substances in physically hazardous situations. Examples: Raoul uses stimulants to help him stay up while driving long distances to see a friend. Patricia drives home after joining friends after work and having several drinks. Since she doesn't feel drunk, Patricia thinks driving is no problem after a few drinks.

**Criterion 9: Use Despite Negative Effects**　　　　☐ **Yes**　　☐ **No**

You continue to use even though you know that a physical, psychological, family, or other problem is likely to occur as a result. Examples: Don drinks despite warnings from his physician that his liver is damaged from years of excessive drinking. Roberta smokes two packs of cigarettes each day despite recommendations from her physician to stop because of chronic respiratory problems.

**Criterion 10(a): Increased Tolerance**　　　　☐ **Yes**　　☐ **No**

You need more of the substance to achieve the desired effect. Examples: John used to get high on two or three drinks. He now often consumes six or more drinks before he feels high. Wanda used to take two tablets of Valium per day. She now takes six and often uses other tranquilizers and alcohol.

### Criterion 10(b): Decreased Tolerance     ☐ Yes     ☐ No

You experience a diminished effect with continued use of the same amount of a substance. Examples: Delinda used to drink a pint or more of liquor every day to feel "the buzz." Now, when she drinks the same amount, she does not feel "the buzz" as before. Alphonso regularly used large quantities of opiate drugs, alcohol, and tranquilizers in the past. Now, when he uses the same quantities, he does not even feel high.

### Criterion 11(a): Withdrawal Syndrome     ☐ Yes     ☐ No

You experience a specific withdrawal symptom when you stop using substances or cut down on the amount you use. Examples: When Michelle stops using alcohol, she becomes nauseous and anxious and has tremors. Russ gets stomach cramps, diarrhea, a runny nose, and goosebumps when he stops injecting heroin or other narcotic drugs.

### Criterion 11(b): Use to Avoid Withdrawal Syndrome     ☐ Yes     ☐ No

You use a substance, and use a similar type (e.g., you substitute Valium for alcohol) to relieve or avoid withdrawal symptoms. Examples: Betty takes tranquilizers constantly because she's afraid she will get sick if she stops taking them. Dean takes a few belts of whiskey in his coffee every morning to quell his shakes and get him settled down so he can go to work. At lunch he has a few drinks to hold him over until after work when he can drink more freely.

*Write the number of symptoms that you checked and rate the severity level*

☐ **2–3 symptoms (mild)**     ☐ **4–5 (moderate)**     ☐ **6 or more (severe)**

## Worksheet 2.2
## Self-Rating Scale

**Instructions:** After reviewing your pattern of substance use and the consequences, rate the current severity of your problem. Then rate your current level of motivation to quit using substances and your confidence level to maintain your sobriety.

### Severity Level of My Problem

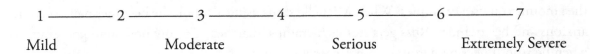

1 ——— 2 ——— 3 ——— 4 ——— 5 ——— 6 ——— 7

Mild            Moderate            Serious            Extremely Severe

### My Motivation Level to Quit Using Substances

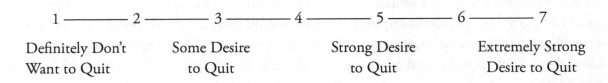

1 ——— 2 ——— 3 ——— 4 ——— 5 ——— 6 ——— 7

Definitely Don't    Some Desire    Strong Desire    Extremely Strong
Want to Quit        to Quit         to Quit        Desire to Quit

### My Confidence in My Ability to Stay Sober

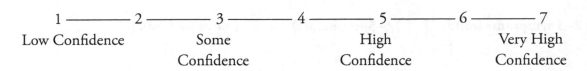

1 ——— 2 ——— 3 ——— 4 ——— 5 ——— 6 ——— 7

Low Confidence      Some          High          Very High
                 Confidence      Confidence     Confidence

# CHAPTER 3 ▸ Recognizing Consequences of Your Substance Use

## Goals

- To understand the consequences of your substance use and its effect on those close to you
- To identify problems caused by your substance use disorder (SUD)

## Harmful Consequences

Substance use can contribute directly and indirectly to problems in any area of your life. SUDs raise the risk of medical, spiritual, psychological, psychiatric, family, and economic problems. Problems may range in severity from mild to life-threatening. Sometimes the effects are subtle or hidden. For example, an attorney initially reported that her work was not affected by her drinking. However, upon closer examination of her drinking patterns and functioning at work, she discovered that her billable hours had decreased by about 15–20% as her drinking worsened. A father of three with a tobacco use disorder didn't think his children were too concerned about his smoking until they told him directly that they were upset, worried, and angry and felt he was cheating them by putting himself at risk for an early death due to smoking.

## Effects of Substance Use Problems on the Family

Alcohol and drug problems often have a negative effect on the family. Loss of family relationships occurs due to separation, divorce, or involvement of child welfare agencies. Families feel neglected, and in some cases their basic needs for food, shelter, and clothing are ignored. The economic burden can be tremendous as a result of spending family income for drugs or alcohol, lost income due to problems caused by substance use, and costs associated with legal, medical, or psychiatric problems. Family members often feel an emotional burden. Anger, fear, worry, distrust, and depression are common. Episodes of neglect, abuse, or violence are often associated with alcohol and other drug problems. SUDs make it difficult if not impossible to function responsibly as a parent or spouse, which leads to problems in family relationships. And, due to the genetic predisposition associated with a SUD, children are vulnerable to developing their own substance use problems. These children therefore need all the help they can get to avoid developing a substance use problem.

## Problems Associated with Substance Use Disorders

Box 3.1 summarizes of some of the more common problems associated with SUDs, as reported in recent publications by the National Institutes of Health and based on our clinical experience. As you can see, these problems occur in all areas of life. After you've reviewed the information in this table, complete Worksheet 3.1: Harmful Effects, at the end of this chapter.

---

**Box 3.1 Problems Associated with Substance Use Disorders**

**Medical and Health:** accidents; injuries; drug overdose; poor nutrition; weight gain or loss; poor personal hygiene; poor dental hygiene, lost teeth, gum disease; increased risk of liver, heart, kidney, or lung diseases; cancers of the mouth or pharynx; gastritis; edema; high blood pressure; sexual problems; complications with menstrual cycle, pregnancy, or childbirth; increased risk for sexually transmitted diseases, HIV, or hepatitis B and C.

---

**Emotional:** anxiety; panic reactions; depression; mood swings; psychosis; feelings of anger or rage; suicidal thoughts, feelings, or behaviors; unpredictable behaviors; aggressiveness; violence; self-harm; feelings of shame and guilt; low self-esteem.

**Work/School:** poor performance; lost jobs or dropping out of school; missing work or school; being undependable and less effective; loss of interest; ruined career; lost opportunities.

**Family:** lost relationships due to separation, divorce, or involvement of child welfare agencies; family distress and conflict; inability to function in parental role or children being raised by relatives or foster care; damaged family relationships; emotional burden on the family (anger, hurt, distrust, fear, worry, depression); poor communication; perpetuation of substance use problems in children.

**Interpersonal Relationships:** lost or damaged friendships; interpersonal conflicts and dissatisfaction; loss of trust or respect of significant others.

**Recreational:** diminished interest in or loss of important hobbies, avocations, or other social or leisure activities.

**Legal:** fines; legal constraints; arrests; convictions; jail or prison time; probation or parole.

**Economic:** loss of income; excessive debts; falling behind in or ignoring financial obligations; loss of security or living arrangements; inability to take care of basic needs for food or shelter; using up all financial resources; inability to manage money; not saving for the future.

## Homework

✎ Complete Worksheet 3.1: Harmful Effects.

## Worksheet 3.1
## Harmful Effects

**Problems Caused by or Worsened by Your Substance Use**

**Instructions:** In the sections below, list any problems that you think were caused by or worsened by your alcohol, tobacco, or drug problem in the past year. Then rank each of the eight categories from the most severe to the least severe, using "1" for the most severe category of problems.

**Medical/physical/dental** _____

_____ _____

_____

**Psychological or emotional** _____

_____ _____

_____

**Work/school** _____

_____ _____

_____

**Family** _____

_____ _____

_____

**Interpersonal relationships** _____

_____ _____

_____

**Recreational** _____

_____ _____

_____

**Legal** _____

_____ _____

_____

**Economic** _____

_____ _____

_____

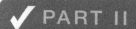

**PART II**

# Change Issues and Strategies

## CHAPTER 4

Treatment Settings for Substance Use Problems

## Goals

- To learn about the different types of professional treatments for substance use problems
- To work closely with your therapist or counselor to figure out your specific goals and what steps you can take to reach them

## Introduction

The American Society of Addiction Medicine (ASAM) outlines levels of care for alcohol or other drug problems in a "stepped care" approach. The ASAM levels are listed here, from the least to most restrictive.

- Level 1: Outpatient treatment
- Level 2: Intensive outpatient treatment and partial hospitalization
- Level 3: Medically monitored intensive inpatient treatment (residential)
- Level 4: Medically managed intensive inpatient treatment (hospital)

You should use the least restrictive level of professional treatment possible unless you have serious medical complications, such as liver disease or gastritis, or serious psychiatric complications such as feeling suicidal, feeling persistently depressed, or feeling paranoid. The sections that follow in this chapter describe the various types of treatment settings and provide some specifics for when each type of treatment is appropriate. Discuss any questions you have about a particular level of treatment with a therapist or a knowledgeable healthcare professional. If you try the least restrictive level of care and find that you are unable to establish and maintain abstinence from alcohol or other drugs, then you should consider a higher level of care and discuss it with your therapist or counselor.

## Levels of Care

### Outpatient and Aftercare or Continuing Care Programs (Level 1)

These programs vary in length from several weeks to months or longer. They may precede or follow detoxification or rehabilitation programs or be used as the sole treatment. Their purpose is to help people achieve and maintain abstinence or reduce harmful substance use, as well as to make personal changes to minimize relapse risk. Individual, group, and family therapy; medication management; and other services may be offered, depending on the specific setting. Outpatient treatment is most suitable if you are not at risk for withdrawal complications and if you have a stable medical and mental condition, show a willingness to cooperate with treatment, are able to maintain abstinence with minimal support, and have a supportive recovery environment. Outpatient treatment can also help you cope with your immediate environmental stresses.

### Nonresidential Addiction Rehabilitation Programs (Level 2)

These short-term (2- to 6-week) programs include intensive outpatient and partial hospital programs. These are appropriate if you do not need the supervision and structure of a residential or hospital-based program. These are sometimes used as "step-down" programs after someone has received treatment in a residential addiction program or hospital-based program or as "step-up" programs when outpatient programs haven't helped someone get or stay sober. These programs are appropriate if you have a minimal withdrawal risk, have no serious medical conditions, have high enough resistance to recovery to require a structured treatment program, are likely to relapse without close monitoring and support, and have an unsupportive environment.

### Inpatient Hospital and Residential Rehabilitation Programs (Levels 3 and 4)

These include both hospital-based and non–hospital-based residential programs. Some are "generic" in the sense that if a person meets the program's criteria, he or she can be admitted to the program. Others are specialized and serve specific populations based on type of and severity of addiction, gender, family status, or ethnicity. The following sections give a brief description of inpatient programs.

### Short-Term Addiction Rehabilitation Programs

Most programs offer a variable length of stay, with many clients staying less than 14 days. Unless you have serious medical or psychiatric problems, non–hospital-based programs are the first choice for rehabilitation. Addiction rehabilitation programs are recommended if you have been unable to get or stay sober through less intensive treatment settings such as outpatient, intensive outpatient, or partial hospital programs. They may also be used if your addiction is of such severity that a period of time in a structured, residential setting is needed to break the cycle of your addiction and help motivate you to establish a foundation for recovery. Short-term rehab programs are also appropriate if you have a high re-lapse potential, if your environment is considered dangerous for recovery, or if you do not have access to outpatient rehabilitation. Rehabilitation programs mainly focus on alcohol and drugs other than tobacco, although some are smoke-free or offer help if someone wants to quit smoking in addition to quitting use of other substances.

### Long-Term Addiction Rehabilitation Programs

If you have a severe pattern of addiction and serious life impairment (e.g., little or no social support, lack of vocational skills, history of multiple relapses, or serious problems with the legal system), you may need a long-term program. A long-term program can help you maintain sobriety by addressing lifestyle and personality issues that you have to change if you are to stay sober over time. Long-term rehab programs include thera-peutic communities, halfway houses, and specialized programs for spe-cific populations such as men, women, women with children, specific ethnic groups, and clients involved with the criminal justice system be-cause of substance-related problems. The trend is toward shorter term programs: therapeutic community programs that once were up to 2 years long now run for several months to less than a year. Due to reduced gov-ernment funding, fewer long-term programs are now available, and they are harder to get into than they were in the past.

Continuing care is important after completing any of these programs. This enables you to continue focusing on recovery issues while you estab-lish a longer period of sustained recovery.

## Detoxification (Levels 3 and 4)

*Detoxification* ("detox") refers to the process of tapering off substance use by using medicine to suppress or reduce withdrawal symptoms. Medical detoxification may be provided in an addiction rehabilitation facility, psychiatric hospital, or medical hospital. Medical detoxification is needed if you have a documented history of addiction, a significant potential for or current evidence of withdrawal complications such as seizures or delirium tremens (DTs), or serious suicidal feelings. A hospital-based program is appropriate if you have concurrent medical or psychiatric disorders that need to be monitored or managed while you detox. Detoxification normally takes up to several days. Detoxification from severe addiction to opioids or benzodiazepines may be started in a hospital or residential program and continued during ongoing treatment in a community setting.

Outpatient detoxification is appropriate if you have a less severe form of substance dependence, you don't show any evidence of serious medical or psychiatric problems, and you have support from family or other significant people. However, be aware that many clinics and doctors do not provide outpatient detoxification.

Detoxification involves monitoring your vital signs and withdrawal symptoms. The detoxification process includes providing medications to prevent or stop physical withdrawal symptoms such as nausea, cramps, runny nose, sleep disturbance, anxiety, and agitation. Rest, nutrition, and evaluation of your physical and mental health are other components of detox. Note, however, that detoxification has limited value if it is not followed by other treatments such as rehabilitation, outpatient care, and/ or participation in mutual support programs.

You should consider being detoxified under medical supervision if you

- Cannot stop using alcohol or drugs on your own without jeopardizing your health
- Have a past history or current medical complications related to withdrawal or the effects of addiction (e.g., DTs, convulsions, elevated blood pressure, gastritis)
- Have a psychiatric disorder (e.g., psychotic symptoms, severe depression, suicidal feelings)

Withdrawal from alcohol or barbiturates is the most dangerous from a medical standpoint. Therefore, it is best that you be evaluated for supervised detoxification rather than quit on your own if you are dependent on these substances. Quitting "cold turkey" can produce serious medical or psychiatric complications, or the discomfort of withdrawal can cause you to continue to use substances to self-medicate your symptoms.

## Other Special Programs

Other specialized treatment programs include those designed specifically for women with children, adolescents, people involved in the criminal justice system, and those with co-occurring psychiatric disorders in addition to a substance use disorder.

### Medication-Assisted Treatment

Methadone maintenance (MM) is used to help individuals with opioid use disorders who have been unsuccessful in their attempts to stop using these drugs. Provided in conjunction with education and counseling services, MM is designed to gradually wean someone from opiates altogether or maintain him or her on a stable dose. A person may remain on MM for months or years. MM helps stop the use of illicit opiates and related criminal behavior and helps recovering individuals function at work and in the community. MM is a helpful treatment if you have been unable to stay off heroin or other opioid drugs despite being involved in other forms of treatment.

Buprenorphine (Subutex, Suboxone, Zubsolv, Bunavail, Probuphine, Sublocade, or generic) is used to help individuals with opioid use disorder in the detox process or as a long-term treatment to reduce opioid use and reduce the risk of relapse. Buprenorphine is being used more and more by addiction treatment programs and physicians but is not available in all treatment clinics because it requires practitioners to get a special waiver from the government. The advantage of buprenorphine over other medications like methadone is that it can be prescribed by office-based physicians rather than having to be dispensed through a treatment center. It is safer in overdose and less likely to be sold on the streets compared to methadone. Naltrexone (Revia and Vivitrol) is another medication that blocks the euphoric effects of opioids. It is another option that you could consider taking to address your opioid use disorder. Narcan is recommended to anyone with an opioid use disorder as a way of reversing a potential drug overdose. Although you do not administer this to yourself, a family member, friend, or other drug user can save your life by administering this drug if you overdose.

## Choosing Your Recovery Goals

Your goals should be based on the severity of your current substance use problem, your motivation to change, and what you want to change about yourself and your lifestyle.

If you are in treatment, you should work closely with your therapist or counselor to figure out your specific goals and what steps you can take to reach them. There may be times when your therapist doesn't agree with your goals. For example, if you have a severe alcohol use disorder and choose the goal of moderating your drinking, your therapist will advise you to work toward abstinence because moderation is not an appropriate goal for you. Or, if you agree to the goal of stopping heroin and cocaine use but still want to use alcohol or marijuana, your therapist will probably advise you to work toward total abstinence because alcohol or marijuana use puts you at risk of returning to heroin and cocaine use.

If you are not sure what goals you want to set for yourself, then your initial goal can be "deciding what I want to change about myself and my alcohol, tobacco, or drug problem." The information in this workbook can help you in that process. Begin by completing Worksheet 4.1: Initial Goals for Treatment.

## Homework

✎ Complete Worksheet 4.1: Initial Goals for Treatment.

**Worksheet 4.1**
**Initial Goals for Treatment**

1. Describe your primary goal for treatment at this time. _____

   _____

   _____

   _____

   _____

2. Describe what specific types of treatment you think you need at this time to reach your goal.

   _____

   _____

   _____

   _____

3. If you have been in treatment before, describe how it helped you. _____

   _____

   _____

   _____

4. What can you do if you feel like leaving treatment before finishing it? _____

   _____

   _____

   _____

## CHAPTER 5

**Motivation and Stages of Change**

## Goals

- To learn the different stages you may go through in your recovery
- To identify the immediate and long-term consequences of either quitting or continuing to use substances
- To learn strategies to increase your motivation for change

Research has identified different stages that you may go through as you change a substance use problem. Although separated for purposes of discussion, you won't necessarily go through all these stages or go through them in an orderly fashion. It isn't unusual to take two steps forward and one step back when changing your alcohol or drug problem. You may get stuck in one stage for a while, go back and forth between stages, or revisit an early stage of change after you have progressed to a later stage. Box 5.1 lists the stages of change. Review this material and then complete Worksheet 5:1: Assessing Your Stage of Change, near the end of this chapter.

## Strategies to Develop Your Motivation

One way to help you accept your problem and develop motivation is to review Worksheet 3.1: Harmful Effects (see Chapter 3). Another way is to complete Worksheet 5.2: Decision-Making Matrix, found at the end of this chapter. The information from these two exercises will help you look at both sides of the issue—quitting or continuing to use. This information

## Box 5.1 Stages of Change

1. The first stage of changing a substance problem, called *precontemplation*, is one in which you aren't aware of your problem. You are resistant to change because you don't think you have a problem. You are not able to admit that you have an alcohol or drug problem even if other people can see it.

2. The second stage is called *contemplation*. During this stage you acknowledge that you have a problem with alcohol or drugs, and you plan to take action within the next 6 months or so.

3. *Preparation*, the next stage, involves planning to do something about your alcohol or drug problem within the next month. You usually let others know about the change you are going to make. Even though you want to change, you still have mixed feelings about it—part of you wants to quit using alcohol or drugs, and part of you doesn't. Don't expect your motivation to be 100% at this point in the change process. You begin to think about the advantages of change.

4. The next stage, *action*, involves changing your alcohol or drug problem. You make a commitment to stop drinking alcohol, smoking, or using drugs. If you are physically addicted and cannot stop using on your own, or if you have a history of complications associated with stopping (e.g., seizure or suicidal thoughts or feelings), you should consider detoxification or hospitalization to help you stop using. In addition to getting sober or clean, during this stage you being to learn more about yourself so that you can also change your thinking, emotions, and self-image. You learn that coping with your substance use problem requires a lot more than simply stopping your use. You address the "nuts and bolts" issues of recovery, such as coping with thoughts about and cravings for substances; dealing with people, places, and things that can influence you to use again; coping with upsetting feelings; and dealing with family and relationship problems. You may become involved in a mutual support program or other forms of social support to build structure into your life and help you stay connected to others who care about your recovery.

5. *Maintenance*, or relapse prevention, is the next stage of change in which you continue to make positive changes in yourself and in your lifestyle. You work hard to prevent a return to alcohol or drug use and accept that there are no easy or quick solutions to your substance use problem. You learn to identify and manage relapse warning signs and high-risk situations. You work on balancing the various areas of your life so that you increase your chances of feeling good about yourself.

Adapted from Prochaska, J. O., Norcross, J. C., & DiClemente, C. C. (1994). *Changing for good.*
New York: William Morrow.

will help you clarify immediate and long-term consequences. Don't be surprised if you discover that you can make a strong case for continuing to use substances as well as a strong case for quitting. It's not a black-and-white issue that is easily resolved because, no matter what problems your alcohol or drug use has caused, you have gained something from using. At first, most people are ambivalent about totally quitting; part of them wants to quit and another part wants to continue drinking or using drugs. Your job is this: look at all sides of the issue, figure out the pros and cons of quitting, and work toward making a stronger case for quitting.

If your motivation wavers after you've been in recovery for a while, figure out what is happening at that time. Share your feelings and experiences with your therapist, an Alcoholics Anonymous (AA) or Narcotics Anonymous (NA) sponsor, other members of support groups, or a confidant who you trust. Consider the following strategies to increase your motivation:

- Renew your commitment to recovery by reviewing your reasons for quitting alcohol or drug use.
- Remind yourself that low motivation is a temporary situation and things can change in the future.
- Review the benefits you have experienced in your recovery so far.
- Identify additional benefits from continued participation in recovery.
- Remember the problems caused by your use of alcohol or other drugs.
- Think about your children or other important people in your life and what your recovery means to them.
- Ask for input from others in recovery to find out what they did during periods of low motivation.

## Homework

- ✎ Complete Worksheet 5.1: Assessing Your Stage of Change.
- ✎ Review Worksheet 3.1: Harmful Effects, which you completed in Chapter 3.
- ✎ Complete Worksheet 5.2: Decision-Making Matrix.

# Worksheet 5.1
## Assessing Your Stage of Change

Answer the following questions to help you determine where you are in your change process. Remember, progress is any movement through one stage to the next. Aim for change, not perfection! Place a check mark (✓) in the appropriate box for each question.

| | Absolutely Yes | Probably | Not Sure | Absolutely Not |
|---|---|---|---|---|
| **Precontemplation/contemplation stages** | | | | |
| 1. Do you think you have a problem with alcohol, tobacco, or other drugs? | ☐ | ☐ | ☐ | ☐ |
| 2. Are you clear about why you want to quit using substances? | ☐ | ☐ | ☐ | ☐ |
| **Preparation stage** | | | | |
| 3. Are you willing to make a commitment to quit using within the next month? | ☐ | ☐ | ☐ | ☐ |
| 4. Do you know what steps to take to stop using on your own? | ☐ | ☐ | ☐ | ☐ |
| 5. Do you need to be detoxified from alcohol or other drugs to stop using? | ☐ | ☐ | ☐ | ☐ |
| 6. Have you told others (family, friends, etc.) about your desire to change your problem with alcohol or other drugs? | ☐ | ☐ | ☐ | ☐ |
| **Action stage** | | | | |
| 7. Do you have a strong commitment to quit alcohol or drugs and stay sober? | ☐ | ☐ | ☐ | ☐ |
| 8. Do you need to change people, places, or things to help you stay sober? | ☐ | ☐ | ☐ | ☐ |
| 9. Do you need to learn to control your thoughts and cravings for substances? | ☐ | ☐ | ☐ | ☐ |

| | Absolutely Yes | Probably | Not Sure | Absolutely Not |
|---|:---:|:---:|:---:|:---:|
| 10. Do you need to address the effects of your substance use on your family or other relationships? | ☐ | ☐ | ☐ | ☐ |
| 11. Do you need to address new ways of dealing with upsetting feelings? | ☐ | ☐ | ☐ | ☐ |
| 12. Are you willing to participate in a mutual support program or other form of social support? | ☐ | ☐ | ☐ | ☐ |

**Maintenance stage**

| | Absolutely Yes | Probably | Not Sure | Absolutely Not |
|---|:---:|:---:|:---:|:---:|
| 13. Do you know the warning signs of a potential relapse and have strategies to help you cope with these **before** you use alcohol, tobacco, or other drugs again? | ☐ | ☐ | ☐ | ☐ |
| 14. Do you know your personal high-risk factors that make you feel vulnerable to using substances and have strategies to cope with these? | ☐ | ☐ | ☐ | ☐ |
| 15. Do you know what steps to take should you actually go back to using substances following a period of abstinence? | ☐ | ☐ | ☐ | ☐ |
| 16. Is your life generally in balance? | ☐ | ☐ | ☐ | ☐ |

There are no questions about the termination phase because we assume that you would not need this workbook if you were in that phase of change.

# Worksheet 5.2
## Decision-Making Matrix: Pros and Cons of Quitting

**Instructions:** In the sections below, write the pros and cons of quitting and of continuing to use alcohol, tobacco, or other drugs. Provide examples of both immediate and long-term consequences of each decision.

### *To stop using or remain abstinent*

| Immediate consequences | | Long-term consequences | |
|---|---|---|---|
| **Positive** | **Negative** | **Positive** | **Negative** |
| _____ | _____ | _____ | _____ |
| _____ | _____ | _____ | _____ |
| _____ | _____ | _____ | _____ |
| _____ | _____ | _____ | _____ |
| _____ | _____ | _____ | _____ |
| _____ | _____ | _____ | _____ |
| _____ | _____ | _____ | _____ |
| _____ | _____ | _____ | _____ |

### *To continue using*

| Immediate consequences | | Long-term consequences | |
|---|---|---|---|
| **Positive** | **Negative** | **Positive** | **Negative** |
| _____ | _____ | _____ | _____ |
| _____ | _____ | _____ | _____ |
| _____ | _____ | _____ | _____ |
| _____ | _____ | _____ | _____ |
| _____ | _____ | _____ | _____ |
| _____ | _____ | _____ | _____ |
| _____ | _____ | _____ | _____ |

# CHAPTER 6 — How to Use Therapy or Counseling

## Goals

- To learn how to get the most out of your treatment

- To familiarize yourself with behaviors that may have a negative impact on your therapy

## Introduction

There are many different types of therapy and counseling approaches for alcohol, tobacco, and other drug problems. Treatment is most effective when it helps you develop and improve skills for dealing with the challenges and demands of recovery and the problems associated with your substance use. Involving your family in the treatment process can also increase the chances of successful treatment; so can active participation in mutual support programs such as Alcoholics Anonymous (AA) or Narcotics Anonymous (NA).

Usually, the more severe your substance use problem, the more time you need in treatment to gain maximum benefit. For less severe substance use problems, short-term outpatient treatment consisting of fewer than 12 sessions is often effective. For more severe problems, longer time in outpatient treatment may be needed. In some instances, detoxification and/or residential treatment may have to precede outpatient therapy.

To increase the chances for recovery, certain attitudes have proved helpful. Recovery is more about change in yourself—attitudes, values, and behaviors—than it is about alcohol or drugs. In fact, only step 1 of the 12 steps of AA and NA mentions the term "alcohol or addiction." The steps address you—the person—not the substance. Here are some ideas to help you get the most out of your treatment and involvement in recovery:

- *Share your story and history.* It is best to be honest in sharing the details of your personal story of substance use so that the professionals assessing you have a true picture of your problem. This will enable them to make recommendations for your treatment and recovery plan. Sharing your story and history honestly in group therapy sessions and AA or NA meetings is also helpful in recovery. You can get support, advice, and feedback from others in recovery.

- *Develop a trusting relationship with a physician, therapist, or counselor.* This is essential in getting the most out of treatment. Let your therapist or counselor know what bothers you, what goes well, what you like and dislike about your work together, and your problems. Make sure you share the truth about close calls, substance cravings, actual episodes of alcohol or drug use, high-risk situations, or motivational struggles.

- *Keep your appointments.* Keep your appointments and stay in treatment long enough to reap the benefits. Do not create excuses and leave treatment against the advice of the people providing your care. Dropping out early is usually a bad sign and often precedes relapse. Be honest and open up in your sessions. Do not keep secrets, especially if you relapse. Your counselor is there to help you, not judge you. Follow through with the agreements you make with your counselor or treatment group.

- *Stay long enough to benefit from treatment.* Treatment is effective to the extent that you stay long enough to benefit from it. For many, a substance use disorder (SUD) is a chronic condition that requires long-term treatment and/or participation in mutual support programs. Many choose to stay active in AA or NA for years.

- *Get help with motivation when it is low.* Your motivation to stay sober may go up and down in the early months of recovery. You can feel enthusiastic one day, then negative about recovery the next day. You may work hard at your change plan only to find yourself feeling less motivated. Reach out to others for help and support if this occurs.

- *Accept that recovery is an ongoing process.* You will always have to actively work on not using alcohol or drugs and being aware of your problem. Since your problem developed over time, it will not easily or quickly be overcome. Recovery happens gradually, often in small steps. Many people in AA or NA have been involved in these programs for years. They know recovery continues long after they stop using alcohol or other drugs. There are no short cuts. Those who expect quick fixes set themselves up for failure.

- *Acknowledge that recovery can be painful.* It requires an open and honest look at life in relation to alcohol and drug use and how this use has affected you and others. This self-examination may evoke guilt, shame, anger, and disappointment. As recovery progresses and changes are made, the pain decreases.

- *Consider abstinence as your goal.* For more severe SUDs, it is best to consider abstinence as a goal since it is common to transfer addictions or accumulate new ones if you continue to use substances. The need for abstinence is stressed in mutual support programs and in their literature. The "basic text" of NA states in the opening chapter that "we could not successfully use any mind-altering or mood-changing substance." That book, written by individuals recovering from drug addiction, also points out how easy it is to justify legal prescriptions and cautions the person who may need some type of mood-altering substance. This problem is also discussed in books written for those with alcohol use disorders. An entire chapter is devoted to "avoiding chemical mood changers" in the book *Living Sober: Some Methods AA Members Have Used for Not Drinking.* Even if it takes you time to work toward abstinence, this is a step in the right direction, as not everyone is able or willing to accept abstinence at first. However, there are times in which a medication with addictive potential may be needed to treat medical or psychiatric conditions such as pain, anxiety, or sleep difficulties.

- *Make changes in yourself.* Making changes in yourself or your lifestyle is the real challenge of recovery. These changes may relate to your thinking patterns, how you handle emotions, how you solve problems, your relationships to others, and how and where you use free time. Your change plan should be based on your problems and what you want to see different in your life.

- *Consider medications for SUD as a tool in your recovery toolbox.* Medications are used to help people safely withdrawal from addictive substances and to help with their ongoing recovery, such as medication-assisted treatments (MAT) or for addiction to opioids, alcohol, or nicotine. If you have an opioid, alcohol, or nicotine use disorder and have trouble staying sober with therapy or counseling alone, ask your therapist to schedule a medication evaluation.

- *Improve your coping skills.* Learning coping skills to deal with problems resulting from or contributing to SUDs is critical for your long-term success. You may need help in developing cognitive (thinking), behavioral, and interpersonal skills to deal with a range of recovery challenges (e.g., setting goals, managing cravings, managing upsetting feelings, dealing with interpersonal conflict, resisting pressures to engage in substance use behavior, identifying and managing early warning signs of relapse and high-risk factors; see Chapters 7–18) or managing co-occurring psychiatric disorders (see Chapter 20). Developing coping skills involves education, awareness, practice and more practice, and the ability to try new things to cope.

- *Address family issues.* Since SUDs affect the family, discuss with your counselor the impact of your substance use on your family, how to improve family communication and relationships, and which treatment and mutual support services can benefit your family (e.g., counseling, Al-Anon, or Nar-Anon meetings). Involving your family is often helpful to both you and your family (see Chapter 12): you get support from them, and they get a chance to share their story and receive help and support. When families and concerned significant others are involved in treatment, the outcome often improves.

- *Expand your recovery network.* A supportive social network consisting of family, friends, and others in recovery who care about your well-being can help you recover in many ways (see Chapters 13 and 14). Work with your counselor to identify new sources of support so you have a larger recovery network to depend on. If you have difficulty asking others for help or support, work with your counselor to learn ways to reach out and ask others for their support.

- *Attend mutual support group meetings.* Open up and share your problems and struggles with your sponsor or peers in mutual support groups. Learn to ask others with similar problems for their help and support. For example, sharing openly with another member of a support group your strong desire to use alcohol or drugs or a decrease in your motivation to change can help you figure out what to do to maintain your sobriety. Go to meetings regularly, especially in the early months of recovery. Participate in meetings by sharing and asking questions. Do not worry about being judged for anything you share or how you thin, because others with alcohol or drug problems like yours know how hard it can be to change at times or how motivation wavers.

- *Prepare for lapse and relapse.* Learning to spot early warning signs of relapse and take action by identifying your potential high-risk situations can help you reduce your risk of relapse (see Chapters 16 and 17). Since you may not experience a straight path in your recovery, prepare for setbacks and emergencies so you have a plan to quickly address any return to substance use or behavior that could lead you back to using alcohol or drugs.

- *Get help with any psychiatric problem.* Psychiatric disorders are common among individuals with SUDs (see Chapter 20). If you think you may have a problem, ask for an evaluation by a mental health professional.

- *Review your progress frequently, especially in early recovery.* There are a variety of ways to check your progress (see Chapter 19). Are you following your plan to change? Are you using active coping skills to manage the challenges of recovery? Are you able to stop your substance use? Are you able to fight through periods of low motivation to change? Are you making improvements in yourself (how you think, feel, or act) or your life? Progress is not an "all or none" issue and should be measured relative to your problems and treatment goals. Your progress is affected by the severity of your problem, your motivation, and your personal resources.

## Difficulty Asking for Help

Pride, fear, embarrassment, worry, and not knowing how can get in the way of asking for help from others. View recovery as a "we" rather than an "I" effort in which you ask others for help or support when you need it. This can happen on many levels: you need a ride to a meeting, you need advice on how to handle a problem, you need someone to listen to your concerns, or you need someone to talk with about something important. You can seek help or support related to any area of life—your health, emotions, relationships, spirituality, finances, or work. Be direct in your request and try to be as specific as you can in terms of what kind of help and support you need from others. Then, be gracious in accepting the help or support offered. The following list presents some ideas on how to ask for and use help from others:

- Face your fears or reluctance to ask for help and support from others.
- Have a list of people (and phone numbers) you can rely on for help or support.
- Share your concerns and feelings with at least one or two confidants (people you trust).
- Take risks in opening up and sharing with others.
- Attend mutual support meetings or participate in online meetings

## Leaving Treatment Early or Against Medical Advice

Some people stop treatment before finishing their program or course of counseling. Others leave hospital detoxification or rehabilitation programs against medical advice (AMA). The reasons they give for leaving treatment early or AMA are usually smokescreens and not the real reason: the real reason usually relates to a desire to use alcohol or drugs again or lower motivation to finish treatment. One of the features of addiction that contributes to a decision to quit treatment or leave AMA is a "covert" craving. This means that on some level you desire or crave alcohol or drugs, but you attribute your desire to quit treatment to another reason (e.g., you don't like the treatment you're getting, you're not getting the medicine you want, you don't like the staff, you think you know everything taught by the counseling or medical staff, you feel anxious or irritable, or you have some personal business to attend to).

Addiction affects your thinking, emotions, and ability to make decisions in your best interest. If you accept your addiction as an illness or disease and accept that your treatment team or counselor knows more than you about what is in your best interest, you can prevent yourself from quitting treatment early or leaving AMA.

*If you leave AMA, your risk of relapse is higher.* Many people who quit treatment or leave a detox or rehab program use alcohol or drugs right away. It is OK if you want to quit or leave treatment early—just don't do it. Instead, put your desire into words and talk with your counselor, nurse, physician, any other professional involved in your care, an AA or NA sponsor if you have one, or trusted friend or confidant. Sometimes simply putting your desires and problems into words gives these less control over you. If you talk about your addiction, cravings to use, and desire to leave treatment, you may gain a fresh view of what is happening.

## Treatment Outcome

Many studies and surveys of recovery show that participation in treatment, mutual support programs, or both for SUDs is effective, especially if you stay long enough to reap the benefit of it. These positive effects may include:

- Improved rates of getting involved in treatment and recovery
- Improved rates of following your treatment plan and attending your sessions
- Improved rates of completing treatment
- Stopping substance use
- Cutting down on the frequency and amount of substances used
- Improved physical and dental health, and healthcare practices
- Improved mental health
- Improved spiritual health
- Improved family relationships
- Increased satisfaction with intimate relationships and marriage
- Improved financial situation (pay bills, reduce debts, save for future)
- Increased community involvement (volunteer work, voting)
- Improved social behaviors (e.g., fewer problems with the law, improved employment rates, less dependence on welfare)

## Behaviors That Interfere with the Effectiveness of Therapy

Therapy-sabotaging behaviors interfere with getting the most from your counseling or therapy sessions. Being familiar with these behaviors puts you in a position to take action if you experience them. Complete Worksheet 6.1: Therapy-Sabotaging Behavior, to identify behaviors that can impede your progress. After identifying behaviors you have engaged in, think about methods of handling each behavior without letting it interfere with your counseling.

✎ Complete Worksheet 6.1: Therapy-Sabotaging Behavior.

✎ Complete Worksheet 6.2: Review of Your Past Treatment Experiences.

# Worksheet 6.1
## Therapy-Sabotaging Behavior

**Instructions:** Review each behavior below. Place a check mark (✔) next to it if you've ever experienced it in relation to your therapy or counseling. Then, choose two behaviors you have experienced and develop an action plan for coping with each behavior.

— Not attending my sessions on time

— Skipping my session entirely

— Missing sessions because I was upset with my counselor

— Dropping out of counseling after only a few sessions

— Not following through and completing assignments or journal exercises between my counseling sessions

— Blaming my counselor for not helping me enough

— Talking about how to change in my sessions but not actually translating these changes into my life

— Expecting my counselor to solve my problems

— Expecting my counselor to tell me what to talk about in my sessions

— Not opening up and telling my counselor what I really think or feel

— Not telling my counselor when I feel like using

— substances or have actually used between sessions

— Constantly calling my counselor on the phone or leaving messages

— Placing unrealistic demands on my counselor

— Not properly taking medications for an addiction or psychiatric disorder

— Not accepting responsibility for those things over which I have control

— Not accepting responsibility for

_____

(things over which I have influence)

— Blaming others for my behavior choices

— Placing myself in high-risk situations

Behavior 1: _____

_____

Action Plan: _____

_____

_____

_____

Behavior 2: _____

_____

Action Plan: _____

_____

_____

## Worksheet 6.2
## Review of Your Past Treatment Experiences

Check the following types of treatment you have received in the past for your addiction. For each item you check under "Treatment Programs and Counseling or Therapy," write in the number of different times you received this treatment during your lifetime. For each "Medication" you have used, write in how long you took this medication.

### Treatment Programs and Counseling or Therapy

☐ Detoxification: # of times_____
☐ Residential or hospital-based rehab (less than 30 days): # of times_____
☐ Residential or hospital-based rehab (more than 30 days): # of times_____
☐ Halfway House: # of times_____
☐ Therapeutic Community: # of times_____
☐ Partial Hospital or Day Treatment Program: # of times_____
☐ Intensive Outpatient Program: # of times_____
☐ Outpatient Counseling: # of times_____
☐ Program for Women: # of times_____
☐ Program for Co-Occurring Disorders (SUD + Mental Illness): # of times_____
☐ Specialty Program for Criminal Justice Problems: # of times_____

### Medication-Assisted-Treatments

☐ Methadone Maintenance (for opioid use disorder): how long?_____
☐ Buprenorphine (Subutex, Suboxone, Zubsolv, Bunavail, Probuphine, Sublocade for opioid use disorder): how long?_____
☐ Naltrexone (Revia or Vivitrol for opioid use disorder): how long?_____
☐ Disulfiram (Antabuse for alcohol use disorder): how long?_____
☐ Naltrexone (ReVia or Vivitrol for alcohol use disorder): how long?_____
☐ Acamprosate (Campral for alcohol use disorder): how long?_____

1. How many different times have you been administered Naloxone (Narcan) to reverse an opioid drug overdose?

   ☐ 0   ☐ 1   ☐ 2   ☐ 3   ☐ 4   ☐ 5   ☐ over 5

2. How many different times have you left detoxification, hospital-, or residential-based treatment against medical advice?

   ☐ 0   ☐ 1   ☐ 2   ☐ 3   ☐ 4   ☐ 5   ☐ over 5

3. How many different times have you stopped partial hospital, intensive outpatient, or outpatient treatment before it was finished?

☐ 0  ☐ 1  ☐ 2  ☐ 3  ☐ 4  ☐ 5  ☐ over 5

4. Overall, how would you rate your personal investment in treatment *in the past?*

☐ None  ☐ Low  ☐ Moderate  ☐ High

5. Overall, how would you rate your personal investment in treatment *at the present?*

☐ None  ☐ Low  ☐ Moderate  ☐ High

6. Describe how treatment helped you in the past. Be as specific and detailed as you can.

_____

_____

_____

_____

_____

7. If you dropped out of treatment early in the past, or left a program against medical advice, describe the effects of this (on your alcohol and drug use, your health, your relationships, and other areas of your life).

_____

_____

_____

_____

_____

8. What could you do to help yourself if you begin thinking about missing your sessions, dropping out of treatment, or leaving a program against medical advice?

_____

_____

_____

_____

_____

# CHAPTER 7  Overview of Goal Planning

## Goals

- To begin to set and prioritize your recovery goals
- To learn about the different paths and components of recovery

## Introduction

Recovery is a process of change in which you improve your health and wellness. You set goals to work toward stopping substance use and learn skills to change yourself and your lifestyle so you can live substance-free.

There are different paths to recovery. These paths include using individual, group, and/or family therapy; engaging in a treatment "program" such as a residential or nonresidential rehabilitation program; taking medications for addiction to alcohol, opioids, or nicotine; engaging in mutual support programs such as Alcoholics Anonymous (AA), Narcotics Anonymous (NA), or non–12-step programs; participating in chat room discussions or online recovery meetings; using support from other people; and participating in other community or self-growth activities that help you sustain recovery from a substance problem. Some people also use recovery applications to aid their recovery. These are online tools in which you monitor symptoms of a substance use disorder (SUD), behaviors, and potential relapse signs, and you take action to manage the challenges you face in recovery. A recovery application often involves connecting with others in a support system so you can reach out for help when you are struggling with recovery. You may use more than one path to recovery over time based on the severity of your problem and what you find helpful.

Recovery goal planning aids your process of change and involves

- Becoming educated about your substance use problem (e.g., causes; effects on your physical, mental, and spiritual health; effects on your relationships and life; consequences of continued substance use; paths to recovery that can help you; and treatments needed)
- Developing a desire to change and dealing with periods of dips in your motivation to change or follow your recovery plan
- Meeting the demands and challenges of recovery, such as managing emotions, desires, and cravings to use and resisting social pressures to use
- Setting specific goals for change
- Developing action plans to help you change and developing a relapse plan to help you maintain changes

Strengthening your existing coping skills and learning new skills to meet the demands of recovery are essential for long-term change. If you have struggled to sustain recovery from an opioid or alcohol addiction, talk with your counselor or a healthcare professional about the role of medications in recovery (see Chapter 15).

Your recovery plan may address one or several areas of recovery: physical, emotional or psychological, family, social or interpersonal, spiritual, or lifestyle. The specific goals you choose are personal, based on how you see your substance use problem and what you believe you need to change about yourself and your lifestyle. When you finish reading this chapter, complete Worksheet 7.1: Goal-Planning. This will help you begin to set goals and develop action plans to reach your goals. You can come back and add to your Goal-Planning worksheet later, after you have reviewed additional sections of this workbook. You may photocopy the worksheet from this book or download additional copies at the Treatments *That Work* Web site at http://www.oup.com/us/ttw. You can revisit this issue after you've completed all the sections of this workbook that you think pertain to you. Goal planning is an ongoing process: you are always going to be working toward goals and making changes in yourself and in your lifestyle.

### Physical Recovery

The physical component of recovery includes

- Getting alcohol- or drug-free
- Taking care of physical or dental problems resulting from or worsened by your substance use
- Eating a balanced diet to ensure proper nutrition
- Getting sufficient sleep, rest, and relaxation to reduce stress and help increase energy
- Exercising regularly to maintain good physical health and reduce stress
- Managing physical craving to use substances (see Chapter 8)

Stopping substance use offers an excellent opportunity to be more health-conscious and to take better care of your body. Medications can help support your recovery as they reduce cravings.

### Emotional or Psychological Recovery

This component of recovery includes

- Accepting that you have a problem and making a commitment to do something about it
- Developing motivation to change and working through periods of low motivation
- Challenging negative thinking that can lead you back to substance use
- Coping with trauma, upset feelings, stress, and other life problems without resorting to using alcohol, tobacco, or other drugs for relief or escape (see Chapter 10)

If you have a coexisting psychiatric disorder, you will need to address this. However, be careful about attempting to deal with too many issues too soon in the recovery process. Therefore, we advise you to wait until you've had a substantial period of sobriety (at least several months) before attempting to deal with any deep-seated emotional problem such as the impact of physical, sexual, or psychological trauma. The exceptions are (1) if you and your therapist believe you need to address these trauma issues now, or (2) you need to develop a safety plan if you are currently in an unsafe and abusive relationship or if you feel seriously depressed, hopeless, suicidal, or concerned that you might harm someone else. If your psychiatric symptoms are causing significant personal distress or impairment in your life, you need to address these (see Chapter 20).

### Family Recovery

Because loved ones are usually affected in one way or another by substance use problems, it helps to examine how your problem has affected your family. Then you can decide what you can do to improve your relationships with family members. Often, it is helpful to invite them to attend therapy sessions, education groups, or "open" AA or NA meetings. You can also encourage your family to attend support groups such as Al-Anon or Nar-Anon. Some communities have other types of mutual support programs for family members. Taking a close look at your problems' impact on your family may temporarily contribute to feelings of guilt and shame (see Chapter 12). In the long run, however, you put yourself in a better position to develop stronger family ties. A book was added to this series (*A Family Guide to Coping with Substance Use Disorders*) to help families understand alcohol and drug problems, how to support you, and how to engage in their own recovery if needed.

### Social or Interpersonal Recovery

Developing a recovery support system that can help and support you can make your recovery a "we" rather than an "I" process. Your recovery support system can include peers in recovery, family, friends, or other supportive people in the community (see Chapter 13). You can also participate in your community in activities unrelated to recovery as a way of being engaged with others (e.g., volunteer work or being part of a group that shares mutual interests).

Personal relationships and leisure interests are frequently damaged by substance use problems. You may have to make amends to others hurt by your substance use, rebuild damaged relationships, make new friends with others who do not get high, learn to assertively refuse offers to use, and develop healthy leisure interests to replace time spent using substances. If you have a long-standing addiction, you may have to learn to have fun again and find new leisure activities that provide you with a sense of enjoyment and fulfillment.

### Spiritual Recovery

This area of recovery refers to overcoming the feelings of shame and guilt that often accompany a substance use problem. Shame refers to feeling bad about yourself, like you are defective or weak. Guilt refers to feeling bad about the things that you did or failed to do when using substances. For some people, developing a sense of meaning in life is an important component of their spiritual recovery. Belief in a higher power and participation in formal religion are two common ways in which people work on their personal spirituality. As recovery progresses, some find it helpful to "give back" to others suffering from similar problems. Some mutual support programs do not believe in the need for a relationship with a higher power for a successful recovery. Therefore, you may receive conflicting viewpoints on the issue of spirituality in recovery; only you can decide what works for you. Also, many people interpret spirituality from a broad perspective that goes beyond belief in following a specific religion or belief in a higher power. Mindfulness and meditation, for example, are common disciplines used to get in touch with one's inner self.

### Other Areas of Recovery

Areas such as work, school, hobbies, legal issues, exercise, money, and creativity may also need to be addressed in your change plan. For example, if your substance use has caused problems with your job or significant financial problems, you need to deal with these. Surveys of recovery show that paying bills on time, paying off debts, or saving for the future are improvements made by many people. Information about lifestyle balance is presented in Chapter 18. This information can help you plan goals related to these other areas of recovery.

## Prioritizing Your Goals

In addition to having specific recovery goals, you have to set priorities. This involves working on the most pressing issues first. You can sabotage your progress if you work on late recovery issues while ignoring early recovery issues. For example, Darren's drug addiction wreaked havoc on his family, causing his parents to feel worried, angry, and at their wits' end about how to help him. His dependency also damaged many of his other relationships. So that he could eventually try to fix some of the relationship damage, Darren first had to sustain his abstinence and learn to manage his constant cravings to get high. His initial goal was to get totally off drugs. This was followed by learning to manage his cravings and find healthy social support. After he took care of these critical issues, he was in better psychological shape to begin working on developing better relationships with his family and other people.

If you will not or cannot get totally off alcohol or drugs as the first step, think about what steps you can take to move toward change, rather than doing nothing at all and letting your problem get worse. If you start the process now, even if you fight within yourself over whether or not to stop completely, at least you can give yourself a chance to make this decision later. It's OK to admit you don't yet know if you want to change. Use the information in this workbook to help you decide if you want to change your substance use problem.

## Homework

✎ Complete Worksheet 7.1: Goal-Planning.

## Worksheet 7.1
## Goal-Planning

**Instructions:** For each domain of recovery, list any changes you want to make. For each change that you identify, write the steps you can take to help you achieve your goal. Try to be as concrete as you can in identifying your goals and your change strategies.

| Change | Goal | Steps toward change |
|---|---|---|
| **Physical** | _____ | _____ |
| | _____ | _____ |
| | _____ | _____ |
| | _____ | _____ |
| **Emotional or psychological** | _____ | _____ |
| | _____ | _____ |
| | _____ | _____ |
| | _____ | _____ |
| **Family** | _____ | _____ |
| | _____ | _____ |
| | _____ | _____ |
| | _____ | _____ |
| **Social or interpersonal** | _____ | _____ |
| | _____ | _____ |
| | _____ | _____ |
| | _____ | _____ |
| **Spiritual** | _____ | _____ |
| | _____ | _____ |
| | _____ | _____ |
| | _____ | _____ |
| **Other (work, economic, etc.)** | _____ | _____ |
| | _____ | _____ |
| | _____ | _____ |
| | _____ | _____ |

## CHAPTER 8

# Managing Cravings and Urges to Use Substances

## Goals

- To learn strategies that will help you prevent or manage your cravings

- To begin tracking your cravings daily over the next few months

- To identify the things that trigger your cravings in order to plan coping strategies

## Introduction

A *craving*, which can vary in intensity from mild to very strong, is a longing for or a desire to use a substance. Your craving can be a desire for the euphoric high associated with using substances, or it can be a desire to avoid or escape unpleasant moods or physical symptoms such as those associated with withdrawal. An *urge* is your intention to use substances once you have a craving. You can have a strong craving with very little intention to use, or your intention to use can be quite high, making you more vulnerable to relapse unless you use active coping strategies to help you through your craving and urge.

Cravings can be *overt*, so that you are aware of them, or they can be *covert* (hidden from your awareness) and show up in indirect ways such as irritability. Cravings tend to be more frequent and stronger in the early phases of recovery. Individuals addicted to heroin often report intense

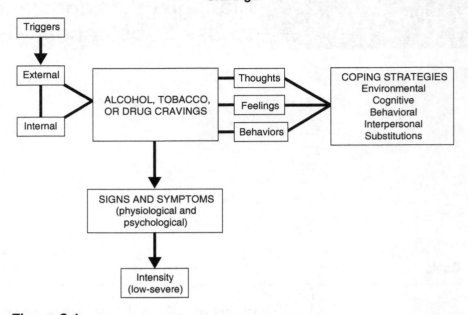

**Figure 8.1**

Craving triggers and intensities.

"drug hunger" that leads them back to using drugs again if they do not find relief.

Cravings for substances are triggered by something external (people, places, events, experiences, or objects) or internal (feelings, thoughts, or memories). Your cravings not only vary in intensity from low to severe, but also in how they show in your thoughts or how they make you feel physically. When you experience a craving, your thoughts and feelings determine how you cope with it. These connections are shown in Figure 8.1 and discussed in further detail in this chapter.

It takes time adjust to not using substances, both physically and mentally. It also takes time to figure out what triggers your cravings and to practice ways of managing them. The strategies reviewed in this chapter should help you prevent or manage your cravings.

## Rating Your Cravings Daily

Learning to identify and label your cravings is the first step toward controlling them. You can call them whatever feels comfortable—urge, craving, desire, need to get high, and so forth. When you start your recovery, track your cravings on a daily basis so that you can see how they change from day to day. It also helps to be aware of how cravings and urges show in physiological and behavioral symptoms. Anxiety, tension, sweaty palms, racing heart, irritability, avoiding people, and lying to people are just a few common ways in which your cravings may show up. Use Worksheet 8.1: Daily Craving Record, later in this chapter, to track your cravings over the next few months. (Figure 8.2 shows an example of a completed Daily Craving Record.) You may photocopy the form from this book or download multiple copies from the Treatments *ThatWork* Web site at http://www.oup.com/ ttw/us. Take a few minutes at the end of each day and rate the average intensity of the cravings you had during the day using a scale of 0 to 5: a rating of 0 indicates no cravings, 1 indicates low craving intensity, 3 indicates moderate craving intensity, and 5 indicates severe craving intensity. Because the first 90 days of recovery present the highest risk of relapse, we recommend that you track your cravings so you can see how the ratings change over time. If you abstain from substances, the intensity of your cravings usually lessens as time goes on. However, there may be days when you experience a temporary increase in your cravings. For example, Sharon's daily ratings were "severe" for the first 2–3 weeks and "moderate" to "severe" during the next 2–3 weeks. The intensity of her cravings decreased during the second and third months. About 6 weeks into her abstinence, she experienced severe cravings for a day. As with any increase in craving severity, the important issue is managing it without using. Eventually, all cravings go away or lessen in severity.

As you track your cravings and rate them daily, pay close attention to the internal and external triggers that you associate with these cravings and the coping strategies you use to avoid taking a substance. For example, Sharon's cravings have recently increased. Sharon has been able to figure out a connection between upset feelings in a relationship and an increase in the severity of cravings. The next two sections will discuss the connection between your cravings, triggers, and coping strategies.

## Identifying Triggers to Use Substances

Identifying the people, places, events, and situations that trigger your cravings or urges helps you anticipate triggers, which can in turn help you plan coping strategies.

## Ratings of Intensity of Cravings

**Instructions:** Each day, use the scale to rate the average intensity (0–5) of your cravings to use alcohol, tobacco, or other drugs.

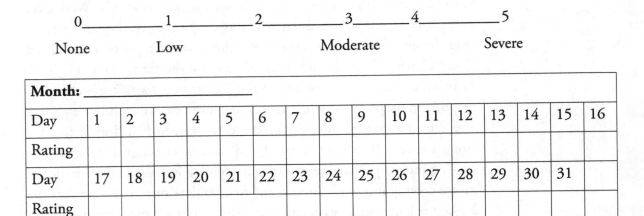

| Month: | | | | | | | | | | | | | | | | |
|---|---|---|---|---|---|---|---|---|---|---|---|---|---|---|---|---|
| Day | 1 | 2 | 3 | 4 | 5 | 6 | 7 | 8 | 9 | 10 | 11 | 12 | 13 | 14 | 15 | 16 |
| Rating | | | | | | | | | | | | | | | | |
| Day | 17 | 18 | 19 | 20 | 21 | 22 | 23 | 24 | 25 | 26 | 27 | 28 | 29 | 30 | 31 | |
| Rating | | | | | | | | | | | | | | | | |

| Month: | | | | | | | | | | | | | | | | |
|---|---|---|---|---|---|---|---|---|---|---|---|---|---|---|---|---|
| Day | 1 | 2 | 3 | 4 | 5 | 6 | 7 | 8 | 9 | 10 | 11 | 12 | 13 | 14 | 15 | 16 |
| Rating | | | | | | | | | | | | | | | | |
| Day | 17 | 18 | 19 | 20 | 21 | 22 | 23 | 24 | 25 | 26 | 27 | 28 | 29 | 30 | 31 | |
| Rating | | | | | | | | | | | | | | | | |

| Month: | | | | | | | | | | | | | | | | |
|---|---|---|---|---|---|---|---|---|---|---|---|---|---|---|---|---|
| Day | 1 | 2 | 3 | 4 | 5 | 6 | 7 | 8 | 9 | 10 | 11 | 12 | 13 | 14 | 15 | 16 |
| Rating | | | | | | | | | | | | | | | | |
| Day | 17 | 18 | 19 | 20 | 21 | 22 | 23 | 24 | 25 | 26 | 27 | 28 | 29 | 30 | 31 | |
| Rating | | | | | | | | | | | | | | | | |

**Figure 8.2**

Example of a completed Worksheet 8.1: Daily Craving Record.

External triggers include people, places, events, situations, or objects that directly or indirectly contribute to your desire to use substances. Common "people" triggers include drinking buddies, drug dealers, partners or roommates who use substances, or coworkers and friends who smoke in front of you. Any place where you previously used substances (e.g., home, office, bar, friend's house, street corner, car) can trigger a desire to use. Similarly, events or situations in which substances are being used can be a trigger for you. These include but are not limited to parties; holiday, religious, or personal celebrations; after-work get-togethers; or business meetings. Even objects can trigger your cravings. These include the sight or smell of alcohol, tobacco, or other drugs; the smell of a particular perfume or cologne; the sight of paraphernalia associated with using (e.g., lighters, mirrors, pipes, papers, needles, alcohol mixers); and the sight, smell, or experience of other objects associated with using. For example, Ryan identified certain pieces of music as triggers for marijuana use. Even when he had no desire to use, if he heard certain songs while riding in the car, he would experience a craving for marijuana. Common triggers for smokers are a cup of coffee and the end of a good dinner, as these are often associated with using cigarettes.

Cravings and urges can also be triggered by internal factors such as feelings, specific thoughts and memories, or physical sensations. Distressing feelings such as anxiety, depression, or anger can also trigger desires to use. It takes time and effort to learn to manage feelings. Negative emotional states are the most common relapse risk factor. Therefore, learning skills to manage your feelings will reduce your vulnerability to relapse. Chapter 10 of this workbook includes strategies for managing your upsetting feelings. Positive thoughts and memories of using can trigger cravings and urges as well. Examples include, "I really don't have a problem," "I can handle a few," "There's nothing like a few drinks (cigarettes, joints, lines of cocaine)," "I can't stand living without getting high on drugs," and "Sex is so much better when I'm buzzed up."

Sometimes, cravings will be random and may happen at any given day or time. At other times, however, cravings may be more likely to happen during specific days or times. For example, when Dana first quit drinking, her cravings were like clockwork: as soon as the "cocktail" hour arrived, her desire for a few drinks before dinner increased. When she ate out in a nice restaurant, she associated having a few glasses of wine with enjoying a good meal.

Although we classify triggers as internal and external for purposes of discussion, they are often interrelated: an external trigger will lead to increased thoughts of using.

Complete Worksheet 8.2: Substance Use Triggers, later in this chapter, to help you identify triggers, the degree of threat each represents, and strategies to help you cope with them. Helpful coping strategies are summarized in the following section.

## Strategies for Managing Cravings and Urges

When possible, choose a strategy that provides a substitute "payoff." For example, if you drank to relax and cope with stress, then you need an alternative way to relax and reduce stress. If you smoked marijuana or snorted cocaine to enhance sex, then you need to find ways to enjoy sex without relying on drugs. If you smoked cigarettes to quell your anger, then you need to find healthier ways of dealing with anger.

As you review the following coping strategies, place a checkmark next to those you have successfully used in the past or can use in the future.

### Environmental Coping Strategies

☐ Reduce environmental cues by getting rid of the substances you are trying to quit using. There is no need to keep cigarettes, alcohol, or drugs in your house if you quit using.

☐ Get rid of paraphernalia used to prepare or ingest drugs (e.g., lighters, ashtrays, needles, mirrors, papers).

☐ In early recovery, when possible, avoid people, places, events, and things that you feel represent a high risk of relapse.

### Cognitive Coping Strategies

☐ Talk yourself through the craving.

☐ Tell yourself that you are capable of coping with a craving no matter how strong it is.

☐ Remember that cravings always pass in time.

☐ Buy yourself time by saying you'll put off using for a few hours.

☐ Remember the troubles caused by using alcohol or other drugs.

- [ ] Ask for help and strength from a higher power.
- [ ] Imagine the craving as a wave that you are surfing to safety. Rather than fighting against the wave, you ride it to shore without getting engulfed in it. "Ride out or surf" the craving and it will eventually leave you.
- [ ] Delay your decision by telling yourself you'll wait until later in the day or tomorrow before you use. By that time, your desire may have decreased in intensity or left completely.

## Behavioral Coping Strategies

- [ ] Distract yourself with an activity.
- [ ] Do something physical, such as take a walk, jog, or work out, to release tension.
- [ ] Write in a journal or complete a daily craving record.
- [ ] Read recovery literature for help and inspiration.

## Interpersonal Coping Strategies

- [ ] Talk to friends in recovery.
- [ ] Talk to family or other supportive people.
- [ ] Go to a recovery meeting and share your cravings.
- [ ] Leave situations immediately if the pressure to use feels too strong to resist.
- [ ] Avoid interpersonal "set-ups." These are relationships or encounters that influence you to use. This influence may be overt or direct, or subtle and indirect. If, for example, you want to date someone who uses alcohol and drugs or have a sexual encounter with someone who is drinking or using drugs, you may not initially feel like using. Later, your desire to use may increase as the situation unfolds and the person you are with invites you to use or uses in front of you.

## Substitute Coping Strategies

- [ ] Smokers find it helpful to chew gum or eat mints or hard candy when they feel like having a cigarette.
- [ ] Substituting a soft drink or other nonalcoholic drink is helpful during times or situations associated with alcohol use, such as during the pre-dinner cocktail hour or a wedding reception.

## Homework

✎ Use Worksheet 8.1: Daily Craving Record, to track your cravings over the next few months.

✎ Complete Worksheet 8.2: Substance Use Triggers, to help you identify triggers, the degree of threat each trigger represents, and strategies to help you cope with them.

# Worksheet 8.1
## Daily Craving Record

### Ratings of Intensity of Cravings

**Instructions:** Each day, use the scale to rate the average intensity (0–5) of your cravings to use alcohol, tobacco, or other drugs.

0 —————— 1 —————— 2 —————— 3 ——— 4 —————— 5

None       Low         Moderate       Severe

**Month:** _____

| Day | 1 | 2 | 3 | 4 | 5 | 6 | 7 | 8 | 9 | 10 | 11 | 12 | 13 | 14 | 15 | 16 |
|---|---|---|---|---|---|---|---|---|---|---|---|---|---|---|---|---|
| Rating | | | | | | | | | | | | | | | | |
| Day | 17 | 18 | 19 | 20 | 21 | 22 | 23 | 24 | 25 | 26 | 27 | 28 | 29 | 30 | 31 | |
| Rating | | | | | | | | | | | | | | | | |

**Month:** _____

| Day | 1 | 2 | 3 | 4 | 5 | 6 | 7 | 8 | 9 | 10 | 11 | 12 | 13 | 14 | 15 | 16 |
|---|---|---|---|---|---|---|---|---|---|---|---|---|---|---|---|---|
| Rating | | | | | | | | | | | | | | | | |
| Day | 17 | 18 | 19 | 20 | 21 | 22 | 23 | 24 | 25 | 26 | 27 | 28 | 29 | 30 | 31 | |
| Rating | | | | | | | | | | | | | | | | |

**Month:** _____

| Day | 1 | 2 | 3 | 4 | 5 | 6 | 7 | 8 | 9 | 10 | 11 | 12 | 13 | 14 | 15 | 16 |
|---|---|---|---|---|---|---|---|---|---|---|---|---|---|---|---|---|
| Rating | | | | | | | | | | | | | | | | |
| Day | 17 | 18 | 19 | 20 | 21 | 22 | 23 | 24 | 25 | 26 | 27 | 28 | 29 | 30 | 31 | |
| Rating | | | | | | | | | | | | | | | | |

**Worksheet 8.2**
**Substance Use Triggers**

**Instructions:** List people, places, events, situations, objects, feelings, thoughts, memories, or times of day that trigger your cravings or urges. Rate the level of threat presented by each trigger using the scale below. Finally, list strategies for coping with each trigger that will help you avoid using.

0 ———— 1 ———— 2 ———— 3 ———— 4 ———— 5

No Threat                    Moderate Threat              Severe Threat

| Trigger (external or internal) | Level of threat (0–5) | Coping strategies |
| --- | --- | --- |
| | | |
| | | |
| | | |
| | | |
| | | |
| | | |
| | | |
| | | |
| | | |
| | | |
| | | |
| | | |
| | | |
| | | |

## CHAPTER 9

# Managing Thoughts of Using Substances

## Goals

- To identify and practice controlling thoughts of using to decrease the risk of relapse
- To learn to use a variety of coping strategies to manage your thoughts of using

## Introduction

Thoughts of using alcohol, tobacco, or other drugs are common. Anyone who stops using a substance will think about it again. It's a normal part of the change process to think about something that you once enjoyed or on which you became addicted. Thoughts of using are often associated with other recovery issues discussed in this workbook, such as cravings, social pressures, family and interpersonal conflicts, and upsetting feelings.

Your specific thoughts can contribute to urges or cravings or to feelings such as depression or anger. Challenging and changing your thoughts can help you stay sober and feel better about yourself and your life. However, like other recovery skills, controlling thoughts of using takes practice. It also requires you to be aware of when your thoughts are getting control of you and your "addictive thinking" is taking over.

Complete Worksheet 9.1: Managing Thoughts of Using, found at the end of this chapter. It lists some of the common thoughts experienced by others trying to quit alcohol, tobacco, or other drugs. Note which ones you've had yourself and add your own thoughts. Then write counterstatements to help you practice new ways of thinking.

## Strategies for Managing Thoughts of Using

You can gain greater control over your thoughts of using substances by drawing on a variety of coping strategies.

- *Monitor your thoughts.* Completing Worksheet 9.1: Managing Thoughts of Using will help you begin the process of monitoring your thoughts of using substances.
- *Devise counterstatements.* After you identify some of your specific thoughts, you can develop counterstatements ahead of time to help you fight off your negative thoughts. In the long run, you will have to learn to create counterstatements as new thoughts arise because you cannot prepare for every thought ahead of time.
- *Don't act on your thoughts.* There is a big difference between thoughts and feelings, and between thoughts and actions. Just because you have a thought doesn't mean you have to act on it. Sometimes all you have to do is ignore your thoughts. Other times, you have to take a more aggressive approach and challenge your thinking or change some of the messages you give yourself in how you think.
- *Remember the benefits of not using substances.* Remind yourself of all the benefits you've already experienced from not using, as well as the benefits you expect to experience if you continue not using. Benefits can be physical, emotional, social, spiritual, or financial. Even small benefits are important, especially in early recovery.
- *Remember the problems caused by using.* Remind yourself of the problems actually caused by past use, as well as problems that may occur if you return to substance use. These problems can be in any area of your functioning or your life.
- *Think through the drink or drug.* Alcoholics Anonymous (AA) and Narcotics Anonymous (NA) advise you to think through the whole process in a rational way so that you see the potential negative outcome of using as well as the potential positive outcome of not using. For example, "I'll feel good and enjoy using, but only for a short time. I'll want more, then will use more. Drugs will control me and what I do. I'll feel guilty for using again. If I fight off this thought and not use, I'll feel good about myself. I know I won't have

to worry about bad things happening. And, I won't have to lie and cover up for my using again. It will be another small victory in my recovery. It will motivate me to continue working my recovery plan."

- *Practice positive affirmation.* Repeat to yourself statements such as, "I can choose not to use," "I'm capable of staying sober," "I control my thoughts; my thoughts don't control me," or "I want to avoid smoking (drinking or using drugs)." Even if you don't feel comfortable saying these affirmations or don't believe them, if you keep repeating them, they may eventually take hold so that you do begin to believe them.

- *Think of yourself as a sober person.* Start each day with the thought that you are sober from alcohol or other drugs. See yourself as capable of getting through another day without using alcohol, tobacco, or other drugs. View this as a normal part of who you are.

## Homework

✎ Complete Worksheet 9.1: Managing Thoughts of Using, to help you practice challenging thoughts of wanting to use and learn new ways of thinking.

**Worksheet 9.1**
**Managing Thoughts of Using**

**Instructions:** Review the list of common thoughts associated with relapse. Add some personal thoughts to the list. Then, list counterstatements and strategies you can use to change these thoughts in order to control them and prevent them from leading to substance use.

| Thoughts | Counterstatements |
|---|---|
| 1. *I'll never use again. I've got my problem under control.* | _____ |
| 2. *A few cigarettes (drinks, lines of cocaine, etc.) won't hurt.* | _____ |
| 3. *I can't have fun or excitement if I don't use.* | _____ |
| 4. *I need something to take the edge off and help me relax.* | _____ |
| 5. *Life is difficult. I need to escape for a while.* | _____ |

| Thoughts | Counterstatements |
|---|---|
| 6. I can't fit in with others if they use and I don't. | |
| 7. What's the point in staying sober? It really doesn't matter. | |
| 8. I'm going to test myself to see if I can have just one. | |
| 9. How can I go out with John if I don't drink? | |
| 10. I'll never get out of debt, I might as well get drunk. | |
| 11. I could drink and no one would ever know. | |

# CHAPTER 10 ▶ Managing Emotions

## Goals

- To learn how upsetting emotions can cause difficulty in your recovery
- To learn the most common upsetting emotional states and strategies for coping with them
- To increase sharing of positive emotions in your life

## Introduction

Upsetting emotions or feelings are among the most common difficulties in recovery. Feelings such as anger, anxiety, boredom, depression, guilt, and shame can contribute to relapse and cause you unhappiness. Mismanaged feelings can cause problems in your relationships and ability to get along with others. An emotion that persists over time is referred to as a *mood*. For example, if sadness continues over time and does not improve, it may lead to a depressive disorder, which is a treatable psychiatric condition.

Many people use alcohol or other drugs to cover up their feelings or make them less painful. However, substances can affect your judgment and exaggerate feelings, making them worse than they actually are. For example, the effects of alcohol or drugs can turn mild irritation or anger into passionate hatred or violence. Under the influence of alcohol, you might inappropriately express simple attraction as unremitting love.

In the section that follows, each of the most common upsetting emotional states is briefly discussed. This chapter concludes with a discussion of practical strategies to manage your emotions. You'll note that there is a lot of overlap among coping strategies regardless of the specific emotions or feelings with which you are dealing. After you read the rest of this chapter, complete Worksheet 10.1: Emotions. Use this worksheet to rate the emotional states you need to address in your recovery. Then use this information to develop your own recovery coping strategies.

## Impact of Emotions on Substance Use

### Anger

Difficulty handling angry feelings is one of the biggest roadblocks to recovery. Two common problems are expressing anger too freely and inappropriately, often in hostile, aggressive, passive-aggressive, or violent ways, or letting it build up inside, avoiding direct, appropriate expression. Both of these extremes contribute to personal unhappiness and strained relationships.

If you "let it all hang out" whenever you feel angry without thinking through the consequences, your goal should be to gain greater control over your expression of anger. You need to think before you act. On the other hand, if you suppress your angry feelings and stew on the inside, you need to give yourself permission to express anger appropriately and to learn healthy ways of sharing your anger with others.

Anger is sometimes labeled as the emotion you feel when underneath it you may feel hurt or disappointed. Even when anger is the second emotion, however, learning to manage it can enhance your recovery. This can make it easier to deal with disappointment or other emotions that you initially label as anger.

### Anxiety

Anxious feelings are common in the early stages of recovery, although for some people anxiety persists for months. Anxiety and worry are two sides of the same coin: anxiety refers to the physical side and shows in sweaty palms, fast heartbeat, or edginess; worry refers to the mental side and shows an excess concern about an event, situation, or relationship. "Anticipatory" anxiety refers to the fear that something might happen.

Worrying about not getting a job before going on a job interview, worrying about being rejected by another person before asking him or her out on a date, and worrying about having a panic attack in public before leaving your house are examples of anticipatory anxiety. Anxiety and worry become serious problems when they lead to serious personal distress or to avoiding people, situations, or events.

If your anxiety and worry persist despite your being sober from alcohol and drugs, cause you personal distress, or interfere with your life, then you may be suffering from a more severe form of anxiety that is a symptom of a psychiatric disorder. You should consult with your therapist and be evaluated to determine if you have one or more of the anxiety disorders. If you have a panic disorder, agoraphobia, or generalized anxiety disorder, you can benefit from treatment by a mental health professional. There are many effective psychological and medication treatments to help you manage an anxiety disorder.

## Boredom and Emptiness

Living without alcohol or drugs can be boring, especially if substance use and related activities were a big part of your life. The "straight" life can seem like a drag at first. You may miss the action of drinking events such as parties; of getting, preparing, or using drugs; or of socializing with others who are drinking or getting high. As recovery progresses, you may become bored with the routine. You may have to relearn how to have fun without alcohol or drugs and redevelop other interests.

When you quit using alcohol or drugs, you may find that you are temporarily bored with your job, your relationships, or how your life is going. Before making any major changes, however, be sure to think through your options very carefully. This type of boredom is different from being bored with your leisure activities or social life. Hasty decisions regarding a job or relationship should be avoided unless they are necessary; as you relearn how to enjoy life without using substances, you may find that an option you considered reasonable earlier would have caused long-term problems.

"Emptiness" refers to feelings of having a void or empty hole in your life since you quit using alcohol or other drugs. Sometimes you don't experience this feeling until you have had several months of sobriety and begin to wonder, "Is this all there is?" You may discover that sobriety is not all that it's cracked up to be and may feel that nothing in your life seems to have much value or meaning for you. Persistent emptiness can be a symptom of chronic depression or borderline personality disorder. Professional treatment—therapy, medications, or both—can help if you have one or both disorders.

## Depression

Depression is frequently caused by the acute and chronic effects of alcohol or other drugs on the central nervous system. When you stop using, depression can result from physical withdrawal or from the psychological trauma of giving up something that was important in your life. You can also experience depressed feelings when you closely examine your life and discover that your substance use caused you a lot of problems and losses. Although feelings of depression may go away after stopping alcohol or drug use, they can represent a high risk for relapse, especially if they are not recognized and dealt with effectively.

With continued abstinence from alcohol or other drugs, most depressions go away in time. However, if your depression persists despite several weeks or months of total abstinence and is accompanied by problems with your sleep, appetite, concentration, energy, or sexual interest; hopeless feelings about the future; or thoughts of suicide or the devising of a suicide plan, then seek mental health treatment immediately. If your current therapist is not qualified to assess and treat your depression, ask for assistance in finding a mental health professional who is. All types of clinical depression can be effectively treated with therapy, medications, electroshock therapy (for more serious levels of depression that may not respond to other treatments), or a combination of these.

## Guilt and Shame

*Guilt* refers to feeling at fault or "bad" about your behaviors—what you did or failed to do. For example, Jerry feels guilty about arguing with his wife, using family money for alcohol, cursing and fighting with his brother when drunk, and getting arrested for driving under the influence. Lavette feels guilty about ignoring her parents and not being available for her children.

*Shame* refers to feeling unworthy or "bad" about yourself—feeling defective, weak, or less than others because of your substance use problem. This was best expressed by Jack, addicted to heroin and cocaine, who referred to himself as a "no-good piece of shit."

Although specific strategies are sometimes needed to cope with a particular feeling, there are common strategies that can be used to deal with upsetting feelings; these include

- *Recognize your emotions or feelings.* Improving your ability to recognize your feelings sets the stage for coping with them. Early recognition helps you catch problems before they build up. For instance, mild anger or depression is easier to deal with than severe anger or depression that has built up over weeks or longer.

- *Accept your feelings.* Accept your feelings as real and for what they are. Don't judge whether a feeling is "right" or "wrong" or "good" or "bad." If you feel something, then it is real to you, and you have to deal with it. The important issue is how you let your feelings affect you and how you manage them. Feelings may represent accurate or inaccurate perceptions of situations, but the feelings themselves are real and are neither "right" nor "wrong."

- *Know the causes of your feelings.* Figure out what's contributing to an emotion. This will help you decide on the best coping strategies. For example, if you feel persistent depression because you are in a primary relationship that is unsatisfying, chaotic, or psychologically abusive, recognizing this problem can improve your depression, especially if you make a decision to do something about it. However, keep in mind that some forms of clinical depression do not need an external reason to trigger them.

- *Challenge your thoughts.* If your thinking is contributing to upsetting emotions or feelings, work on changing how you think and the beliefs that underlie your thinking. For example, if you feel extremely anxious about an upcoming job interview and are telling yourself that you won't get the job, challenge your thinking. Tell yourself, "I will do my best on this interview, which will give me a good chance for the job because I'm well qualified." Practice saying these thoughts—out loud if necessary—to build your confidence and comfort level.

- *Share your feelings with someone you trust.* Sometimes it helps to simply put your feelings into words. Telling a trusted friend or family member, "I feel depressed (furious, anxious, worried, lonely)" can help you feel some relief. Sometimes when you share how you feel, the intensity of the feelings decreases. In addition, you frequently gain a new perspective on what you are experiencing. Putting feelings into words also helps reduce the risk of inappropriately acting on them.

- *Increase your focus on and expression of positive emotions in your life.* Positive emotions such as love, affection, joy, compassion, awe, hope, forgiveness, and gratitude can help offset negative ones and enhance your life. Some experts recommend that you aim for a healthy ratio of three to one of positive to negative emotions. Try to go beyond just experiencing a positive emotion and, when appropriate, express it. For example, you probably feel grateful a lot, but keep this to yourself. Practice sharing gratitude with others or write down and reflect on a few things for which you feel grateful.

- *Build structure in your life.* Structure can help you overcome boredom, which is common in early recovery. Structure can also help reduce depression and anxiety, especially if you participate in pleasant activities. Setting specific times and days for activities and sticking to that structure can help you keep going if you find that you are losing momentum.

- *Use physical or creative activities.* These activities help reduce tension and stress, lower depression and anxiety, release anger, and improve self-image. Sports or exercise or music, reading, writing, art, or other creative endeavors can help you express your feelings.

- *Use inner-directed activities.* Meditation, mindfulness, or prayer can help you cope with negative feelings. In addition to reducing stress, anxiety, and depression, these activities can help you feel more energetic, positive, and reflective. For example, prayer is often helpful in reducing feelings of guilt and shame. Mindfulness helps you focus on the present and pay closer attention to your inner self and the environment.

- *Set goals for yourself.* Having goals provides you with the incentive to work toward something that is important to you. Goals can keep you busy, give you something to look forward to, reduce depression or boredom, and give you more structure in your life.

- *Consider medications for persistent and severe anxiety or depression.* If your severe feelings of anxiety or depression persist despite being alcohol- or drug-free for a month or longer; if they cause you considerable personal distress; or if they interfere with your ability to function, you may have an additional mental health problem that could improve with medication. Many nonaddictive medicines are available to treat mental health problems that do not respond well enough to therapy alone.

## Homework

✎ Complete Worksheet 10.1: Emotions, to identify and rate the emotional states you need to address in your recovery.

✎ Develop your own recovery coping strategies.

## Worksheet 10.1
### Emotions

**Instructions:** For each emotion below, rate the degree of difficulty you have in dealing with these feelings without using alcohol or drugs. Then, choose the two emotions that present the most difficulty in your recovery and identify strategies for coping with them.

0 ——————— 1 ——————— 2 ——————— 3 ——————— 4 ——————— 5

None          Low                          Moderate                    Severe

| Emotion | Degree of difficulty coping with emotion (0–5) |
|---|---|
| 1. Anxiety and worry | _____ |
| 2. Anger | _____ |
| 3. Boredom | _____ |
| 4. Depression | _____ |
| 5. Feeling empty—like nothing matters | _____ |
| 6. Guilt | _____ |
| 7. Shame | _____ |
| 8. Loneliness | _____ |

| Feeling or emotion | Coping strategies |
|---|---|
| _____ | _____ |
| | _____ |
| | _____ |
| | _____ |
| | _____ |
| | _____ |
| | _____ |
| _____ | _____ |
| | _____ |
| | _____ |
| | _____ |
| | _____ |
| | _____ |

### Positive Emotions

List examples of positive emotions you can express more often to other people and how doing so can improve the quality of your life.

## CHAPTER 11

Refusing Offers to Use Substances

## Goals

- To learn about direct and indirect social pressures that can raise relapse risk
- To learn how each social pressure affects your thoughts, feelings (emotions), and behaviors
- To plan and practice how you will cope with social pressures to use substances

## Introduction

One of the biggest and most predictable challenges you face in recovery is resisting social pressures to use alcohol, tobacco, or other drugs. This is especially true in the early months of recovery, when you are just getting used to being sober or not smoking and are not used to refusing offers to use.

After difficulty managing a negative emotional state, giving in to social pressures is the second most common cause of relapse. You will face direct social pressures when others may offer you alcohol, tobacco, or other drugs and try to influence you to use. Some people might even get right in your face and try to make you feel like there's something wrong with you if you don't use with them. This may make you feel uncomfortable or awkward, especially if you want to fit in and be "one of the crowd."

You will also experience indirect social pressures when others around you are using but don't offer you alcohol, tobacco, or other drugs or try to convince you to use. Being at a picnic, family gathering, party, athletic event, or special occasion such as a wedding or holiday celebration, or even just watching a movie, can trigger a desire to use.

You aid your recovery by preparing to manage people, places, events, work, family, or social situations that create pressure to use.

1. Identify the direct and indirect social pressures that you are likely to face.
2. Be aware of how each direct and indirect social pressure affects your thoughts, feelings, and behaviors.
3. Plan and practice how you will cope with social pressures to use substances.
4. Evaluate how you handle each pressure, and change those strategies that don't help you.

Figure 11.1 illustrates the issue of social pressures in recovery.

Pressures or offers to use substances come from many sources. People may directly offer you substances, or you may participate in activities in which substances are used. When others are offering you a substance or are using in front of you, a part of you will likely want to use or fit in. Each social pressure influences how you feel, what you think, and ultimately how you act. Anticipating your unique social pressures puts you in a position to develop and practice positive coping strategies.

Although you can avoid many pressures, you cannot avoid them all. Therefore, it helps to plan different strategies you can use to successfully cope with direct and indirect social pressures to use. The key to staying substance-free is having strategies to handle people, places, events, and situations that you are not able to avoid.

Complete Worksheet 11.1: Social Pressures, found at the end of this chapter, to help you identify people, places, and situations that create pressure for you to use substances. After you have identified these pressures, you can develop coping strategies.

## Strategies to Resist Offers to Use Substances

The following list is a summary of coping strategies to help you identify and resist offers to use substances:

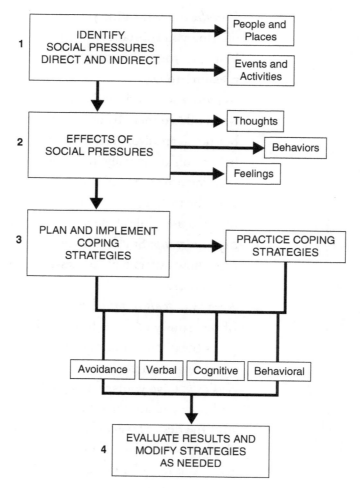

**Figure 11.1**

Social pressures.

- *Awareness.* Be aware of the direct and indirect social pressures you are likely to face. Pay careful attention to thoughts and feelings generated by various social pressures. Also, be aware of situations in which you are setting yourself up to use. For example, trying to quit alcohol but going to a bar to socialize and trying to quit cocaine or marijuana but attending parties at which others use drugs are examples of "set-up" situations. In set-up situations, your risk of using substances rises considerably.
- *Acceptance.* A part of you may always be tempted to give in to pressures to use. Learn to accept and live with this as it is not likely to go away completely. Usually, the part of you that wants to use is strongest in the first few weeks and months after you stop using.
- *Avoidance.* When possible, avoid high-risk people, places, situations, and events, especially when you feel vulnerable to the influence of others or your own desires to use are strong.

- *Visualization.* Imagine yourself in situations in which others are offering you substances. Visualize yourself confidently say NO. Visualize yourself in control of the situation and resisting all pressures to use.

- *Assertiveness.* Clearly and directly state your intent to not use substances when offered them by others. Assertiveness involves being forthright but not aggressive. Practice saying "no" in a direct and assertive manner before you are actually in situations in which others pressure you to use. Practice with your therapist, a trusted friend, family member, or alone by looking in the mirror. You can practice assertively refusing offers to use while alone in your car, at home, or at work.

- *Support group.* Stick with your sober support group. You will learn how others have successfully resisted social pressures to use substances.

- *Keep your goals in mind.* Remind yourself of your sobriety goals and of the gains you've made so far. Regularly review your short-term goals (next few minutes to next few days) and how they fit in with your long-term goals.

- *Self-talk.* Give yourself a pep talk about why you want to stay sober and how you are capable of resisting pressures to use. Talk yourself into the desired way of thinking. Don't allow yourself to fall for the thought, "A few won't hurt." Instead, tell yourself, "I don't need to use; I can resist." Do a quick review of the problems your substance use has caused in your life and the benefits of continued sobriety.

- *Emergency planning.* Some situations can't be avoided, so know your options before a difficult situation occurs. For example, if it is important to attend a social or work event at which alcohol is being served or people are smoking cigarettes, plan to stay only a short time or take a supportive friend with you who knows you are trying to avoid drinking or tobacco use. If you feel the pressure to use mounting in a particular situation, leave immediately. Avoid long discussions about why you don't want to stay or why you aren't drinking or smoking unless you think this will make it easier for you not to use.

## Homework

✎ Complete Worksheet 11.1: Social Pressures.

# Worksheet 11.1
## Social Pressures

**Instructions:** List specific direct or indirect social pressures to use alcohol, tobacco, or other drugs that you expect to face. For each social pressure you list, use the scale below to rate the degree of difficulty you believe you will have in coping successfully with that pressure. Finally, list coping strategies you can use to cope with these social pressures.

0 ——————— 1 ——————— 2 ——————— 3 ——————— 4 ——————— 5

No Threat                 Moderate Threat         Severe Threat

| Social pressures | Degree of difficulty (0–5) | Coping strategies |
|---|---|---|
| | | |
| | | |
| | | |
| | | |
| | | |
| | | |
| | | |
| | | |
| | | |
| | | |
| | | |
| | | |
| | | |
| | | |
| | | |
| | | |

## CHAPTER 12

Dealing with Family and Interpersonal Problems

## Goals

- To identify and address conflicts in your family and interpersonal relationships
- To examine your usual style of relating to others
- To begin to formulate and use strategies for resolving your conflicts

## Introduction

Problems and conflicts in family and interpersonal relationships are common in recovery and can contribute to relapse if you don't have a plan to deal with them. Conflict, tension, and disagreements are normal parts of human relationships. Not addressing these head-on sets you up to feel angry, frustrated, and unhappy. Therefore, take some time to review the important relationships in your life. See if any of these relationships have serious problems or conflicts and examine what is causing these problems. Then you can begin to formulate strategies to resolve your interpersonal conflicts.

Sometimes interpersonal problems are obvious. For example, Art became angry at his wife for embarrassing and insulting him in front of friends at a dinner party. Helen felt hurt and sad when her husband "forgot" her birthday. Curt and Kathy argue over money, sex, the children, and other issues, which causes bad feelings toward each other. They feel their marriage is on the verge of collapsing.

In contrast, interpersonal conflicts are sometimes subtle, covert, or hidden. In some instances, you may have an idea that something isn't quite right in a relationship. For example, Megan and her sister Jan seldom plan activities with both of their families, believing that everyone is too busy. On another level, Megan knows deep down that there is an unspoken tension between the two families. Although she has never said this directly to her sister, Megan does not like or respect Jan's husband and feels uncomfortable being around him. Her discomfort plays a major role in minimizing contact between the two families. In other instances, you may be unaware that anything is wrong unless you think long and hard about your relationships with family members. For example, Juan seldom visits his parents, who live within a few hours' drive of his house. Juan and his parents seldom call each other on the phone. The accepted excuse is, "Everyone is busy." However, after further exploration, Juan admitted that he feels angry because every time he visits home, his mother complains nonstop about his father, and his father is hard to be around because he's moody, critical, and not sociable. It also bothers Juan that his parents seldom make any attempt to visit his family and don't take much of an interest in the lives of his three children.

## Listening to Experiences of Family Members

It is common for family members to experience hurt or pain as a result of a loved one's substance use problem. Your family is probably no exception. This is especially true if your substance use has led to physical or verbal abuse; unpredictability; irresponsibility in your role as a spouse, parent, or family member; inability to meet the emotional or financial needs of your family; or serious medical problems. Complete Worksheet 12.1: Family Effects, to help you identify how your family has experienced your substance use problem.

Although it can be painful, it is important to hear from your loved ones what it has been like for them. This requires you to be patient, able to listen without being defensive and making excuses for your behaviors, and willing to accept the emotional pain of family members. Some recovery programs recommend "making amends," a process in which specific steps are taken to reduce the damage caused by a substance use problem (review steps 8 and 9 of Alcoholics Anonymous [AA] or Narcotics Anonymous [NA] with a sponsor or counselor). The form that making amends takes can vary from one person to the next. Making your recovery a high priority, involving your family, and listening to their experiences are ways to start the "making amends" process.

## Social and Work Relationships

Other relationships can be negatively affected by substance use problems. You may have taken advantage of, lied to, manipulated, ignored, used, or abused your friends or work associates. For example, Serena often had coworkers cover for her and do part of her job when she came in late for work after attending parties the night before. Alexi, a college professor, failed to do his share of committee work on a special project for his department, causing other faculty members to feel angry and let down. He often missed meetings, giving several poor excuses why he didn't do his share of the work on time.

Complete Worksheet 12.2: Relationships, to help you begin to address specific problems you are having with others. Also, complete Worksheet 12.3: Interpersonal Style, to help you examine your usual style of relating to others. You can use this worksheet to help you determine if there are things you need to change in how you relate to others. (All of the Chapter 12 worksheets can be found at the end of this chapter.)

## Strategies to Improve Your Relationships

The following list presents strategies to help you deal with interpersonal problems and conflicts, as well as improve your relationships with family members and other important people in your life.

- *Identify interpersonal conflicts and problems.* Be aware of your relationship conflicts and problems. Then you can prioritize and work on the one or two that are most important. Remember, these conflicts can be obvious or hidden.
- *Know your role in these conflicts.* Avoid the trap of blaming your problems on others. It usually takes two to have a problem. Conflicts are often caused less by specific events that occur than by your interpretation of these events and your interpersonal style. For example, if you are too aggressive, you need to tone down your aggression. On the other hand, if you are too passive and feel

victimized by others, you need to learn to assert yourself more. If your interpersonal style creates problems in your relationships, work with your therapist to make changes in how you relate to others.

- *Face your conflicts directly.* Interpersonal conflicts usually don't go away on their own, and nothing is accomplished by ignoring them. Deal with your conflicts head-on and avoid the tendency to wish them away or to allow too much time for conflicts to build even more. Maintain control over the expression of your feelings and behaviors when you are discussing conflicts with another person. Accept that conflicts are a normal part of relationships and may provide an opportunity to make relationships better in the long run. There are some couples, however, who seldom express conflict toward each other yet do well in their relationship; it is as if they have an agreement "not to disagree" about anything or enter into critical or conflictual interactions.

- *Express your feelings directly.* Healthy relationships require an ability to share feelings with others. This includes upset feelings such as anger or disappointment as well as positive feelings such as love or appreciation. Many people have an easier time sharing upsetting feelings than positive feelings. However, make sure you express gratitude, love, and other positive feelings toward those closest to you. How you express your feelings is very important. It helps to pay close attention to your tone of voice, facial expressions, body movements, and choice of words. For example, you can tell a loved one in a nonjudgmental and matter-of-fact way that you are angry, implying that you want to communicate and resolve differences, or you can communicate anger in a hostile and negative way that will push the other person away and cause the situation to get worse.

- *Involve your family in recovery and in your life.* When possible, involve your family in some of your treatment sessions and invite them to attend self-help meetings such as Al-Anon or Nar-Anon. There are many advantages to family involvement in your recovery: your family can gain a greater understanding of what it's like for you to stop using substances, provide you with support, and share their feelings and experiences. This sometimes leads to family members becoming involved in a recovery program themselves to deal with their own feelings and issues. If you are heavily involved in mutual support groups, pay close attention to your family, too, so that you don't focus all your attention on your recovery and ignore their needs.

- *Encourage your family to share.* Ask those close to you to share their experiences related to your substance use and behavior so that you gain a greater understanding of their perspectives. Be prepared, however, to hear some unpleasant things. Family members and close friends often see the worst side of substance use problems and your behaviors.

- *Deal with family members or close friends who use illicit drugs.* Avoid being around family members or close friends when they are using illicit drugs. Let them know that you are quitting and that it's too difficult to be around them when they use drugs. If your spouse or partner uses drugs, you will face a special stress and will need to figure out how best to deal with it. Whether or not the relationship can continue while you work on your recovery depends on factors such as how long you've been together, how committed you are to each other's welfare, how realistic it is to be in an active relationship and stay drug-free when your partner gets high, and whether your partner is willing to get help or work together so both of you can stay drug-free.

- *Deal with family members or close friends who smoke or drink.* If you feel too much pressure being around family members or friends who smoke cigarettes or drink alcohol, even if they don't smoke or drink excessively, then you should minimize the time you spend with them when they are smoking or drinking. You can leave such situations entirely if you worry that you might relapse. It also helps to let those who are close to you know that you are trying to quit using alcohol or tobacco. If they visit your house, it is your right not to have alcohol available. It is also your right not to allow anyone to smoke in your house. Letting people know ahead of time makes it easier for them to accept your way of dealing with smokers and drinkers in your house.

- *Deal directly with your partner if he or she drinks excessively.* If your spouse or partner clearly has an alcohol problem, it will be more difficult for you to stay sober if he or she drinks in front of you. If your spouse or partner refuses to quit or get help for the drinking problem, then you need to evaluate the relationship to determine if it is too stressful for your recovery. For family members or friends who drink excessively, it is far better to suggest that they get help for themselves rather than to preach about why they should stop drinking.

- *Admit your mistakes.* If you make a mistake in one of your important relationships, don't dwell on it. Instead, admit it to the other person and try to avoid making the same mistake again.

- *Compromise.* Mutual relationships require the ability to give and take, or compromise. You must be able to give in at times, even when you feel your position is right. What might be "right" for you individually might not be "right" for the relationship. For example, Brianna sometimes gives her adult daughter, Lilly, money because Lilly manages her budget poorly. Brianna's husband Nathan does not agree with his wife giving their daughter money, but understands and accepts his wife's position because not helping their daughter creates too much stress and worry for his wife. Compromise also involves doing things with others that you might not particularly enjoy. You do these things because the other person is important to you.

- *Nurture your important relationships.* The best and most satisfying relationships are those that are actively nurtured by positive action. One way of nurturing a relationship is to consciously do and say positive things that the other person will appreciate. In this way, you not only work on problems, but you also work on growth in your relationship.

- *Seek family counseling if problems persist.* If you are unable to resolve specific problems in your family or significant relationships despite trying some of the ideas just discussed or participating in mutual support programs, seek family or relationship counseling.

## Homework

- Complete Worksheet 12.1: Family Effects.
- Complete Worksheet 12.2: Relationships.
- Complete Worksheet 12.3: Interpersonal Style.

## Worksheet 12.1
## Family Effects

**Instructions:** List your family members. Then describe ways in which the behaviors related to your substance use problem have affected each family member.

| Family member | Behaviors/consequences of my substance use |
|---------------|---------------------------------------------|
| _____ | _____ |
| _____ | _____ |
| _____ | _____ |
| _____ | _____ |
| _____ | _____ |
| _____ | _____ |
| _____ | _____ |
| _____ | _____ |
| _____ | _____ |
| _____ | _____ |
| _____ | _____ |
| _____ | _____ |
| _____ | _____ |
| _____ | _____ |
| _____ | _____ |
| _____ | _____ |
| _____ | _____ |
| _____ | _____ |

## Worksheet 12.2
## Relationships

**Instructions:** Describe the problematic relationships in your life. Write about what you can do to improve these relationships.

| Problem | Ways to improve problem |
|---------|-------------------------|
|         |                         |
|         |                         |
|         |                         |
|         |                         |
|         |                         |
|         |                         |
|         |                         |
|         |                         |
|         |                         |
|         |                         |
|         |                         |
|         |                         |
|         |                         |
|         |                         |
|         |                         |
|         |                         |
|         |                         |

# Worksheet 12.3
## Interpersonal Style

**Instructions:** Following is a list of statements about interpersonal style. Circle the number that corresponds to the extent to which each statement describes you. Then complete the two items below the list of statements.

|  | Doesn't describe me | | Somewhat describes me | | Definitely describes me | |
|---|---|---|---|---|---|---|
| 1. I say what I think or feel to others and don't hold anything back. | 0 | 1 | 2 | 3 | 4 | 5 |
| 2. I worry about hurting others and hold on to my feelings. | 0 | 1 | 2 | 3 | 4 | 5 |
| 3. I lash out at others when I'm upset or mad at them. | 0 | 1 | 2 | 3 | 4 | 5 |
| 4. I regularly share positive feelings with others. | 0 | 1 | 2 | 3 | 4 | 5 |
| 5. I often criticize others a lot and express negative feelings. | 0 | 1 | 2 | 3 | 4 | 5 |
| 6. I have trouble talking to strangers. | 0 | 1 | 2 | 3 | 4 | 5 |
| 7. I consider myself to be shy and have trouble opening up to others. | 0 | 1 | 2 | 3 | 4 | 5 |
| 8. I relate easily to others and like meeting new people. | 0 | 1 | 2 | 3 | 4 | 5 |
| 9. I let other people close to me know what's important to me. | 0 | 1 | 2 | 3 | 4 | 5 |
| 10. I don't like to argue with others and avoid arguments when I can. | 0 | 1 | 2 | 3 | 4 | 5 |
| 11. I let people take advantage of me too easily. | 0 | 1 | 2 | 3 | 4 | 5 |
| 12. I consider myself to be an aggressive person. | 0 | 1 | 2 | 3 | 4 | 5 |
| 13. I consider myself to be an assertive person. | 0 | 1 | 2 | 3 | 4 | 5 |

| | Doesn't describe me | | Somewhat describes me | | Definitely describes me |
|---|---|---|---|---|---|---|
| 14. I consider myself to be a pushover and a passive person. | 0 | 1 | 2 | 3 | 4 | 5 |
| 15. I avoid situations where I have to talk in front of other people. | 0 | 1 | 2 | 3 | 4 | 5 |
| 16. I use alcohol, tobacco, or other drugs to help me socialize with others. | 0 | 1 | 2 | 3 | 4 | 5 |

Identify one aspect of your interpersonal style that you want to change.

_____

_____

List several steps you can take to help you change this behavior.

_____

_____

_____

_____

## CHAPTER 13

Building a Recovery
Support System

## Goals

- To learn the benefits of having a recovery support system
- To identify people and organizations who can provide you with support
- To work to overcome any barriers to asking for help
- To learn strategies for creating and using an effective recovery support system

## Introduction

Many people in recovery from a substance use disorder (SUD) find it beneficial to use the support of other people or organizations. You can expand your support network by overcoming any reluctance you have in reaching out for help and support from others, identifying key people or organizations that can support your recovery, and taking an active role in making your recovery more of a "we" than an "I" process so you do not rely only on yourself.

## Benefits of a Recovery Support System

A *recovery support system* consists of people and organizations that provide you with help and support in your efforts to stop using alcohol, tobacco, or other drugs. A positive support system is associated with a better outcome and has many benefits. It enables you to gain from the strength, hope, experience, and advice of others who care about your recovery. You can lean on others during difficult times as well as share your triumphs and the positive goals that you achieve. You can also share mutual interests or activities with people in your support system.

Many people find it helpful to approach recovery from a "we" instead of an "I" perspective. Although self-reliance is helpful in long-term recovery, in the early stages, reliance on others can make a big difference in whether or not you use alcohol or other drugs.

As we discuss in Chapter 14, mutual support programs and recovery clubs can play a critical role in your recovery. You can benefit from the fellowship of these programs as well as from the specific recovery approach such programs take.

Complete Worksheet 13.1: Recovery Network, at the end of this chapter. This worksheet will help you identify people and organizations who can provide you with support. It will also help you see the potential benefits of specific people and organizations.

## Barriers to Asking for Help and Support

Although a recovery support network is helpful, you may find it hard to ask others for help and support. This may be due to shyness, fear, guilt over your previous behavior, lack of self-confidence, poor social skills, or a belief that you should be able to handle your own problems, that you are not worthy of others' efforts to help you, or that others will reject you if you seek their support. Another barrier is choosing the wrong people to ask for support. These include people who won't understand or accept your interest in staying off alcohol or other drugs or who believe you must be out of your mind for wanting to stop.

Once you identify barriers that will interfere with your ability to ask others for support, you can then work on overcoming these barriers. For example, Tina identified being shy and being fearful of rejection as her major barriers to asking for help. She worked with her therapist to practice initiating conversations with others. After successfully testing this out over time, Tina then worked on requesting help and support from other members of Alcoholics Anonymous (AA). She dealt with her fear of rejection by examining what evidence she had that others would reject her. In fact, Tina discovered that there was only a single case of another person having rejected her, and it so happened that this person was notorious for being antisocial and hard to get along with. Tyrone identified pride and excessive self-reliance as his barriers to asking for help. A star athlete who always played a major role on the team, he was not used to being in a position of asking for help from others. When he came to believe that his self-reliance wouldn't be threatened by reaching out for help, he took the risk. Tyrone feels the risk paid off because he was able to benefit from the experiences of another athlete who had overcome a drug problem. This connection helped Tyrone stay focused on his academic and athletic goals and deal effectively with his problem.

## How to Ask for Help and Support

When you choose the right people, there's a very good chance they will respond favorably to your request for help and support. Ask for what you want directly and specifically. When possible, include peers in recovery as part of your support system since they are also working at sustaining long-term recovery and can share their experiences and successful coping strategies with you. Consider the following examples:

"Frank, I'm interested in your being my sponsor. I really like what you've done with your recovery and your straightforward approach to telling it like it is."

"Marie, I quit smoking cigarettes and I'm asking that when you come to my house for dinner next weekend, if you feel like smoking, please do it outside on the porch. Even smelling smoke makes me want to light up, so I appreciate you understanding this request."

"Dad, I finally accepted that my drinking was a serious problem, so I'm on the wagon. I won't be serving any liquor at Tim's graduation party and hope you are OK with this."

"Lynn, I'd like to go with you to some Narcotics Anonymous (NA) meetings. I'm nervous about going by myself and would enjoy your company."

"David, I really enjoyed it when we worked out in the past. I'm changing some bad habits and going back to the gym. I would like to get back into running and working out with you."

"Melissa, I know you kicked cigarettes a couple years ago. I can't take my work breaks with the others who smoke now. Do you mind if I join you sometime during break time so my temptation to smoke isn't so bad?" "Fran, I want to get high so bad I can almost feel the drugs going into my veins. Instead of copping drugs, I stopped at a gas station and I'm calling you instead of chasing drugs, like you suggested during a recent talk we had. Can we meet to talk so I stay on track with my recovery?"

## Strategies to Develop a Support Network

The following is a list of strategies to help you develop and effectively use a recovery support system:

- *Identify supportive people.* Know who you want to be involved in your network. Consider how they can help and how and when you can ask them.
- *Ask for help directly.* When you make a request for help and support, be as specific as you can. Face your reluctance to ask for help and take a risk. Practice ahead of time what you will say if you think this will make you more comfortable and more likely to follow through with making a specific request. Also, if you choose people who were upset and hurt by your substance use problem, be sure to make amends first (see Chapter 12) to reduce some of the bad feelings that may still exist.
- *Get involved in organizations.* In addition to mutual support organizations specifically related to recovery, think about religious, community, social, or athletic organizations. Being active in organizations can increase your sense of connection to others and provide opportunities to learn from others and participate in leisure, athletic, political, creative, or religious activities.
- *Be active.* If you are in a recovery organization, make a point of talking to someone else in the program at least once a day, especially in the early weeks and months of recovery. Keep at list of at least five names and phone numbers of others in recovery.
- *Face your excuses for resisting help.* Everyone has reasons why he or she cannot ask for help and support, even if he or she believes it could be helpful ("Yeah, but . . . "). Figure out what your excuses are. Consider the following examples:
"I know the others who are trying to quit smoking like me will be glad to talk to me, but I don't want to bother them."
"I know getting a sponsor can help me stay off cocaine, but what if

I pick someone who isn't working a good program?"

"I know I should tell my parents I don't want to be around them
when they are drinking, but I don't want to hurt their feelings."

- *Focus on pleasant activities, not just recovery issues.* If you belong
to a recovery program, find out about enjoyable social events
and activities that the program sponsors or that other members
participate in. Do something fun regularly.

## Homework

✎ Complete Worksheet 13.1: Recovery Network.

**Worksheet 13.1**
**Recovery Network**

**Instructions:** (1) Identify how hard it is for you to ask others for help and support. Then, (2) identify people and organizations that you believe can be a vital part of your recovery network. (3) List the potential benefits of having these individuals and organizations as part of your recovery.

**Describe how difficult it is for you**
**to ask others for help or support**

| People/organizations | Potential benefits |
| --- | --- |
| | |
| | |
| | |
| | |
| | |
| | |
| | |
| | |
| | |
| | |
| | |
| | |
| | |
| | |
| | |
| | |
| | |

# CHAPTER 14 — Mutual Support Programs and Recovery Clubs

## Goals

- To learn about the different types of mutual support programs available
- To determine which type of program may work for you

## Introduction

Numerous mutual support programs exist to help you cope with your substance use problem. The most common of these programs are Alcoholics Anonymous (AA), Narcotics Anonymous (NA), and other 12-step programs. All mutual support programs involve people with alcohol or drug problems helping each other. Whereas some people maintain lifelong involvement in mutual support programs, others use them for a limited period of time. Some people go in and out, using mutual support programs whenever they feel the need. After reading this chapter, complete Worksheet 14.1: Mutual Support Program, at the end of this chapter, to help you determine the potential benefits of a mutual support program. A list of organizations, including their web sites, is included in the Helpful Resources Appendix at the end of this workbook.

Although programs vary in philosophies and approaches, most involve the following:

- *Fellowship*. People with similar problems help each other deal with their alcohol or drug problems. They do this by sharing experiences in and out of meetings, "sponsoring" newcomers (commonly done in AA and NA), and being available to talk about recovery issues of mutual concern, such as how to deal with cravings to use, how to recover from a lapse or relapse, and how to undo the damage inflicted on family members or other people as a result of substance use.

- *Recovery meetings.* These involve discussing recovery issues or listening to personal stories of others who share their experiences with substance use and recovery.
- *Program steps or guidelines.* These involve particular steps you can take to deal with your alcohol or drug problem. Programs such as the 12 steps of AA and NA are seen by many as a way of life, not just a way of overcoming a substance use problem.
- *Recovery literature.* Many booklets, books, and recordings are available to provide you with information, inspiration, and hope. Many are written by people in recovery.
- *Social events.* Some programs such as AA or NA sponsor social events such as holiday celebrations or activities. These events provide an alcohol- and drug-free environment in which you can have fun, meet other people, and not feel pressured to use substances.
- *Internet resources.* Many organizational and individual web sites, blogs, and social media posts provide information about recovery and offer strategies to manage a substance use disorder (SUD). Some web sites include recovery applications that allow you to engage interactively in activities aimed at strengthening your recovery.

## 12-Step Programs

### Alcoholics Anonymous and Narcotics Anonymous

AA, NA, and other 12-step recovery programs are available at no cost to any person who wants to stop drinking or using other drugs. These programs are based on the premise that members can help each other recover from substance use problems. These are the largest and most accessible of all the mutual support programs, with meetings held throughout the world. Many are smoke-free meetings so you do not have to worry about inhaling secondhand smoke from cigarettes smoked by others.

AA and NA view alcoholism and drug addiction as diseases that have physical, psychological, social, and spiritual components. Recovery is a process that addresses these different areas in the 12 steps of recovery, in the other aspects of AA and NA such as discussion or lead meetings, or between "sponsor" and "recovering member." Members help each other by exchanging phone numbers, attending meetings together, providing support to one another, and celebrating positive accomplishments in recovery.

Within AA and NA, there are a variety of "specialty" meetings. These include meetings for those new to recovery, gays or lesbians, business executives, young people, healthcare professionals, those with co-occurring psychiatric illness, and others.

A major component of 12-step programs is reliance on a "higher power" for help. Although many people find this acceptable and helpful in their recovery, others are uncomfortable with anything related to spirituality or religion. You have several options if this part of the program makes you uncomfortable: use only the aspects of the 12-step programs that you are comfortable with philosophically, find other mutual support programs—such as Self-Management and Recovery Training (SMART)—that don't emphasize the need for a higher power (see the Appendix for information), or approach the issue of a higher power with an open mind to see if any aspect of this recovery component can help you.

### Smokers Anonymous and Nicotine Anonymous

These programs adapt the 12 steps for smokers. Similar to all 12-step programs, these focus on not only stopping the behavior (i.e., smoking), but also on making changes in yourself and your lifestyle to help you stay off cigarettes or nicotine.

### Dual Recovery Anonymous

This program is similar to AA and NA, with the main exception that its members are recovering from dual problems of substance use and psychiatric disorders. The 12 steps have been modified to accommodate the psychiatric illness.

### Other 12-Step Programs

Numerous other 12-step programs exist for drug addiction and other life problems. These include Emotions Anonymous, Emotional Health Anonymous, Gamblers Anonymous, Overeaters Anonymous, Sex

Addictions Anonymous, Spenders Anonymous, Sex and Love Addicts Anonymous, and others.

## Other Mutual Support Programs

There are other mutual support programs as alternatives to AA and NA. Each program has a specific philosophy, approach to recovery, meeting format, and written literature. Some of these more common programs are Rational Recovery, SMART Recovery, Women for Sobriety, Men for Sobriety, Alcoholics Victorious, and Moderation Management (MM). Most of these programs help people quit substances and stay alcohol- or drug-free. The exception is MM, a controversial program developed for individuals who don't have a physical dependence on alcohol. MM is not recommended for anyone who has serious physical or psychiatric problems caused or worsened by alcohol use, or for anyone taking medications that interact with alcohol. MM is not a "controlled drinking" program and is intended for problem drinkers, but not for chronic drinkers. MM has a nine-step program of recovery that aims to help the person moderate alcohol use.

The main problem with these alternative programs is that there are a limited number of meetings available and no meetings at all in some areas. Also, some treatment programs and professionals recommend mainly the 12-step programs of AA or NA.

Some of these programs offer online meetings or chat rooms where you can interact with others recovering from a substance problem. Also, there are recovery "applications" that can be used on a computer, smartphone, or other electronic instrument. These applications help you monitor cravings, mood, and other areas of life, give you suggestions; and help you stay focused on recovery.

## Recovery Clubs and Clubhouses

Some areas have recovery clubs or clubhouses for people in recovery. These provide an alcohol- and drug-free environment in which you can attend recovery meetings or other social events. Many offer the chance to informally chat with others in recovery and develop new, sober relationships. You can check with a counselor or other professional who provides treatment for SUDs, or you can ask members of mutual support programs about local clubs. You can also use an internet search engine to ask if there are local "recovery clubs" for addiction, SUDs, or alcohol or drug problems.

## Using Mutual Support Program Resources

You can help yourself in several ways.

- *Become educated.* Read about various mutual support programs and recovery clubs or clubhouses available in your area. Materials can be purchased in bookstores, through the organization that sponsors these programs, or at local meetings. Some materials can be downloaded—some at no cost, others you pay for.

- *Consider your options.* Once you have found out what mutual support programs are available in your area, consider the pros and cons of each program that appeals to you. You don't have to agree with a particular program's philosophy to gain something from it. Don't ask yourself, "Will I like it?" but rather, "How might it help me?"

- *Keep an open attitude.* Many people have unrealistic ideas about how mutual support programs work or what goes on in them. For example, some believe they have to stand in front of a crowd of strangers and confess that they are an alcoholic or a drug addict. You don't usually have to talk unless you want to.

- *Consider previous experiences.* Review your previous involvement, if any, in mutual support programs or recovery clubs or clubhouses to figure out what was most helpful and unhelpful. Even if a particular program wasn't helpful in the past, that doesn't mean it cannot help you now. On the other hand, if you've really tried a program only to find you didn't benefit from it, then try another type of program.

- *Try several meetings.* Attend up to a dozen different meetings before you make a final decision as to whether or not a self-help program can help you. It's hard to judge by just a few meetings because meetings can vary in content and in how they are conducted. You may feel more open-minded at some meetings than at others.

- *Get a meeting list and names of contacts.* Ask your therapist for a list of meetings in your area or consult the phone book or internet for phone numbers. If you are uncomfortable going to meetings by yourself, ask your therapist for names of people who might go with you, ask another person in recovery to go with you, or call the local office or the organization and ask for a temporary sponsor.

- *Develop contacts.* Get a list of telephone numbers of other group members and learn to reach out for help and support. If you have trouble asking for support from others, ask your therapist to help you learn ways of asking for help.
- *Find something beneficial.* Rather than focusing on what you don't like about a particular program or meeting, find something positive, no matter how small. It is your responsibility to find something from the program or meeting that can help you.
- *Establish a support group.* Find a group of people you like and feel a connection with, regardless of the group philosophy. The connections with others who have similar problems can be as beneficial as or even more beneficial than the group philosophy.

## Homework

✎ Complete Worksheet 14.1: Mutual Support Program.

# Worksheet 14.1
## Mutual Support Program

**Instructions:** Complete the following items to help you decide how mutual support programs could help you stop using alcohol, tobacco, or other drugs and help reduce the chances of relapse.

1. Describe what it is like for you to ask others for help and support.

   _____

   _____

   _____

   _____

2. Summarize your previous experiences in mutual support programs (pro and con).

   _____

   _____

   _____

   _____

3. List potential drawbacks of participating in mutual support programs.

   _____

   _____

   _____

   _____

4. List potential benefits of participating in mutual support programs.

_____

_____

_____

_____

5. Which specific mutual support or online program(s) do you think would benefit you in quitting or staying off alcohol, tobacco, or other drugs?

_____

_____

_____

_____

# CHAPTER 15 — Medications for Substance Use Disorders

## Goals

- To learn about types of medication that aid recovery from a substance use disorder (SUD)
- To understand the reasons why some people may have problems with medication
- To learn about withdrawal symptoms and medications that help
- To understand the effects of drug and alcohol use on psychiatric medications
- To determine whether or not you need medication to help with you substance disorder

## Medications for Substance Use Disorders

Medications can help you safely and comfortably withdraw from substances such as alcohol, opiates, or sedatives if you have a physical addiction. The medicines used will depend on the drug or drugs on which you are dependent. Medication-assisted treatment (MAT) is the use of medications approved by the US Food and Drug Administration (FDA), in combination with counseling and behavioral therapies, to provide a "whole-client" approach to the treatment of opioid, alcohol, or tobacco use disorders.

## Opioid Use Disorders

Three medications are used to treat opioid use disorders

1. *Methadone* (Methadose and Dolophine) is an opioid full agonist (an agonist is a drug that activates opioid receptors in the brain and does not block other opioids while preventing withdrawal). This is dispensed only in specialty regulated clinics.
2. *Naltrexone* (Revia and Vivitrol) is a nonaddictive opioid antagonist (an antagonist causes no opioid effect and blocks the effects of other opioids) and is dispensed as a daily pill or monthly injection.
3. *Buprenorphine* (Subutex without naloxone; with naloxone: Suboxone, Zubsolv, Bunavail, and generic) is a partial opioid agonist (meaning it activates the opioid receptors in the brain but to a much lesser degree than a full agonist, and it blocks other opioids while reducing withdrawal risk). It is dispensed as a dissolving tablet, cheek film, 6-month implant under the skin, or monthly injection.

## Alcohol Use Disorders

Disulfiram (Antabuse), acamprosate (Campral), and naltrexone (Revia, Vivitrol) are the most common medications used to treat alcohol use disorder. None of these medications provides a cure for the disorder, but they are most effective in people who work a recovery program. These medications can help reduce craving and the risk of relapse.

## Tobacco Use Disorders

There are three medications approved by the FDA to treat tobacco use disorders (smoking, chewing, or sniffing tobacco):

1. *Nicotine replacement medications* (NRTs) include chewing gum, transdermal patch, nasal sprays, inhalers, and lozenges; they assist with reducing nicotine withdrawal symptoms including anger and irritability, depression, and anxiety. Some of these medications are available over-the-counter.
2. *Bupropion* (Zyban), a medication originally approved as an antidepressant, has also been found to help people quit smoking.

3. *Varenicline* (Chantix) is a nicotine partial agonist that reduces the craving for cigarettes and has been helpful in stopping smoking. Bupropion (Zyban) and varenicline (Chantix) are prescription medications.

## Attitudes About Taking Medication

One of the problems you may face is the pressure from others in recovery not to take any medications. Some misguided people have the wrong attitude about "medications." They think these are the same as "addictive" substances and do not see their potential benefits. This is especially true of methadone, a medication that has helped many people remain drug-free while improving their lives. Remember, other people are entitled to their opinions, but you have the right to take medications to help you in your recovery from an addiction to alcohol or other drugs by adding a tool in your recovery toolbox.

There are several attitude problems you may face yourself regarding medication. First, you have to accept that medications for a SUD or for a psychiatric illness are different from substances used to get high or to self-medicate negative emotional experiences. You are taking medications to treat a disorder and get better. You should not feel guilty for taking medication or believe that it is a "crutch" or that you are "weak" for needing it. Some people resent the idea that they have to take a medicine for a substance use or psychiatric disorder. They argue with doctors, therapists, and family members. Some even refuse medicine altogether or take it for only a short time and then stop. Discuss with your support system your feelings and thoughts about medications and have an open mind about their role in your recovery. You can make an informed decision by being educated about their impact on your recovery. Ultimately, it is your decision whether you choose to take such medications or not.

A second problem is the desire to stop taking medication once your symptoms are under control and you feel better. *Never stop your medications unless you first talk this over with your therapist and doctor.* Many people relapse to addiction or psychiatric illness after they stop or cut down on their medication following a period in which they feel better. Just as you shouldn't stop taking medications for high blood pressure, diabetes, or other medical conditions on your own, you should not stop taking medications for an addiction or psychiatric disorder without first talking to the people taking care of you. Any desire to stop on your own should first be discussed with your doctor, therapist, or counselor, or your Alcoholics Anonymous/Narcotics Anonymous (AA/NA) sponsor if you have one. Another person can help you examine your "real" reasons for wanting to stop taking medications.

A third problem is side effects from medication. If you are having unpleasant side effects that don't go away, call your doctor to ask if your medicines need to be changed or if you need to do something to offset these side effects. Some side effects go away in time. Others become more tolerable over time.

A fourth problem is feeling frustrated that your symptoms are not improving as much as you would like. Some individuals do not respond to certain medications as well as others do. They may try several different types of medication over a period of time and feel frustrated if they don't quickly find the medication that works for them. You have to be patient if this happens. We have observed that many people addicted to opioid drugs who undergo detoxification become impatient when their symptoms do not improve as quickly as they would like. They sometimes make poor decisions and leave a detoxification program against medical advice as a result. Medications aren't equally effective with everyone who has the same symptoms.

A fifth problem is expecting medications to make all of your symptoms or problems go away. While medication can control or reduce symptoms, some chronic or persistent symptoms may remain with you. You have to learn to live with these as best you can. Also, medications cannot take away problems in your life. That is why medications should be used with therapy and/or participation in mutual support programs such as AA or NA.

## Withdrawing from Addictive Drugs

If you have a physical addiction to alcohol or other drugs and have been unable to quit on your own, or if you have a history of complications related to withdrawal—such as seizures, delirium tremens (DTs), severe depression, psychotic symptoms, or suicidal feelings—you should seek medical treatment to help you through the withdrawal process. Medications can reduce, stop, or prevent withdrawal symptoms. Professionals who help you through the withdrawal process can also help you find the type of treatment you need for ongoing help with your addiction since detox in and of itself has little value if not followed by other treatment.

### Alcohol Withdrawal

Withdrawal symptoms usually start on the first day and peak on the second or third day after a person completely stops or significantly cuts down alcohol use after drinking heavily for several days or longer. Symptoms include tremors of the hands, tongue, and eyelids; nausea and vomiting; weakness; sweating; elevated blood pressure or tachycardia; anxiety; depression or irritability; and low blood pressure when in an upright position. More severe cases of withdrawal may include delusions (false beliefs), hallucinations, seizures, or agitated behavior. Alcohol withdrawal can last several days and may be helped by taking benzodiazepines such as diazepam (Valium), chlordiazepoxide (Librium), or oxazepam (Serax).

### Depressant Withdrawal

Heavy or prolonged use of other depressant drugs such as sedatives and tranquilizers can cause withdrawal symptoms similar to alcohol withdrawal symptoms. Withdrawal from depressant drugs is done by gradually tapering off the drug the person is addicted to or by substituting a drug that is similar in its action on the central nervous system. Withdrawal from some of the longer acting tranquilizers takes more than a few days.

### Opioid Withdrawal Syndrome

Symptoms of withdrawal from heavy, prolonged use of opioids include runny nose, tearing eyes, dilated pupils, goosebumps, sweating, diarrhea, yawning, mild hypertension, tachycardia, fever, and insomnia. Symptoms start 6–12 hours after the last drug dose, peak on the second or third day, and usually end within 7–14 days, depending on the specific drugs used and the length of the addiction. Medically supervised withdrawal from opiates or narcotics involves taking methadone (Methadose, Dolophine), buprenorphine (Subutex, Suboxone, Zubsolv, Bunavail, or generic), clonidine (Catapres), or lofexidine (Lucemyra).

### Cocaine and Stimulant Withdrawal Syndrome

Depressed mood, fatigue, disturbed sleep, and increased dreaming are symptoms that sometimes occur during withdrawal from heavy, prolonged use of stimulant drugs. Although there are no severe physical withdrawal symptoms associated with addiction to cocaine or stimulant drugs, medications may be used to help someone through the withdrawal process. Many medications have been studied in the treatment of cocaine and other stimulant addiction. While there is some benefit to these medications, none has been effective.

### Tobacco Withdrawal Syndrome

Symptoms of nicotine withdrawal usually begin within hours of stopping or significantly reducing tobacco use after heavy, regular use. These symptoms include tobacco cravings, irritability, anxiety, concentration problems, restlessness, headaches, drowsiness, and gastrointestinal disturbances. Gum, transdermal patches, nasal sprays, inhalers, and lozenges (NRTs) can be used to help gradually withdraw from use of tobacco products such as cigarettes. Nicotine gum helps to minimize nicotine withdrawal symptoms and to decrease the risk of relapse in the early weeks and months of being tobacco-free. However, the gum can be addictive and should not used if the person has medical conditions such as a recent myocardial infarction, vasospastic disease (impaired arterial blood circulation), cardiac arrhythmia, esophagitis, peptic ulcers, or inflammation of the mouth or throat. Some people complain of side effects such as hiccups, nausea, jaw irritation, and bad taste. A nicotine patch can help stop withdrawal symptoms by decreasing tension, anxiety, irritability, restlessness, and nicotine cravings. The patch gradually releases nicotine into the system, usually over a period of 24 hours. Patches can be used up to several weeks or longer to help a person withdraw from nicotine. Nicotine nasal sprays and nicotine inhalers are two other approaches to decreasing people's urge to smoke.

## Medications to Aid Recovery and Reduce Relapse Risk

### Alcohol Use Disorders

Disulfiram (Antabuse) is a drug used by some people to help "buy time" when they want to drink. Disulfiram will stay in your system for a week or longer, so if you decide to drink, you have to wait for disulfiram to clear your system to avoid getting sick. If you ingest any alcohol while disulfiram is in your system, you will get sick because disulfiram interrupts the body's normal process of metabolizing alcohol. The idea behind this drug is simple: it is supposed to deter you from using any alcohol, but if you do drink and get sick, the punishment will deter you from drinking in the future. Disulfiram usually is recommended only for the short term (6 months or less) due to its effects on the liver. Also, a fatal reaction between alcohol and disulfiram can occur, so it is not recommended if you tend to act impulsively.

Naltrexone is an opioid antagonist that blocks the euphoric effects of opioids, and it is also used with alcohol use disorders. Known by the trade name ReVia as a pill or Vivitrol as a monthly injectable form, naltrexone appears to block the effects of the body's own opioids, which reduces the reinforcing properties of alcohol and thus the desire to drink. Acamprosate (Campral) can help you maintain abstinence from alcohol after you become sober. It appears to lessen the craving to drink alcohol.

### Opioid Use Disorder

Some people who become addicted to heroin or other opioids have an extremely difficult time staying drug-free even though they have participated in rehabilitation or other treatment programs. Opioid agonist therapies with methadone or buprenorphine reduce the effects of opioid withdrawal and reduce cravings. They have been shown to increase retention in treatment and reduce risk behaviors, such as using opioids by injection, that lead to transmission of HIV and viral hepatitis B and C. Medication-assisted treatment with extended-release injectable naltrexone (Vivitrol) reduces the risk of relapse to opioid use and helps control cravings.

### Stimulant Use Disorders

There are no medications with FDA approval to treat stimulant use disorders. Several medications that have been marketed for other disorders show some promise in reducing cocaine use. Among them are disulfiram (Antabuse), modafinil (Provigil), bupropion SR (Wellbutrin SR), desipramine (Norpramin), and topiramate (Topamax). Researchers are also exploring a vaccine to be tested in humans. Some of the medications mentioned earlier, such as bupropion SR and modafinil, have been studied to treat methamphetamine dependence with no success.

### Cannabis Use Disorder

Currently, the FDA has not approved any medications for the treatment of cannabis use disorder, but research is active in this effort.

## Medications for a Coexisting Psychiatric Disorder

If you suffer from a psychiatric disorder in addition to your substance use problem, you may benefit from the use of medications. Psychiatric medications such as antidepressants sometimes have the added benefit of reducing desires to use substances such as alcohol. You should be aware that some psychiatric medications, such as tranquilizers and sedatives, can be addictive and lead to relapse to substance use.

Sometimes, well-meaning counselors or members of 12-step groups take an "all or none" view of medications and take the position that no medication used to change moods is necessary. Remember, anyone can offer you an opinion, but only a qualified physician or other professional is in the position to know whether medications help with a particular psychiatric condition.

## Effects of Drug and Alcohol Use on Psychiatric Medications

Using alcohol, illicit drugs, or other nonprescribed medications can have a negative effect on antidepressant medications by causing the level of medication in your blood to increase or decrease. Even small amounts of alcohol or other drugs can have a negative effect on medications. In some instances, mixing medications with alcohol or drugs can cause serious complications with psychiatric symptoms.

Substance use can also lower your motivation to comply with psychiatric medications. Many people complain that their medication does not work, yet they continue using alcohol and drugs. If you continue to drink or use drugs, do not expect to get the maximum benefit from medications. Also, be aware that some doctors may not prescribe psychiatric medications unless you agree to abstain from substances.

## How to Know If You Need Medication

You should discuss any questions about medications with a therapist or physician who is knowledgeable about recovery from SUDs. Medications can help your ongoing recovery if

- You have been unable to stay off alcohol, opioids, tobacco, or other drugs for longer than a few months at a time
- You have tried other forms of treatment and still go back to using alcohol, opioids, tobacco, or other drugs
- You feel it is difficult not to drink, use opioids, tobacco, or other drugs, although you know you should quit and you want to quit
- You often feel overwhelmed by cravings and strong desires to use alcohol, opioids, tobacco, or other drugs
- You have a lot to lose if you relapse, such as an important relationship, a job, or your professional status or license
- Your physical health or mental stability has been greatly affected by your substance use and will continue to get worse if you use
- You believe medications will help you benefit more from therapy or mutual support programs
- You have an opioid addiction and worry about a drug overdose (this refers to having Narcan available to reverse a potentially fatal drug overdose)

Sometimes, questions are raised about the risks and side effects of medications. Discuss these questions with a physician and with your therapist so that you can do a cost-benefit analysis (Box 15.1). Usually the risks and costs of taking medications are small in comparison with the risks of continued use of alcohol, tobacco, or other drugs.

## Medication-Seeking Behaviors

Some people look for a "magic" medication that will cure their psychiatric illness or addiction and make everything better for them. They think that anytime their symptoms worsen or new ones develop, some pill will magically take these symptoms away, or they hope that a medication can make them feel better when they have serious problems at work or in their

## Box 15.1 Questions to Ask Your Doctor About Medications

1. What is the purpose of this medication?
2. When should I take this medicine, should it be taken with food, or should I avoid eating right before or after taking it?
3. How long will it take for medications to have an effect on my symptoms, and which symptoms are most likely to be relieved?
4. How will I know if this medication isn't working for me?
5. What are the side effects, will they go away, and, if they don't go away, what can I do about these, and which should I report immediately to my doctor?
6. What are the risks of not taking this medication?
7. How long will I need to take medication?
8. What happens if I drink alcohol or use other drugs while I'm taking this medication?
9. Are there other medicines, including over-the-counter drugs, that interact with this medication?
10. What are the dangers of missing dosages of medications or taking more than prescribed?
11. If I feel like quitting my medications, what should I do before stopping?

relationships. Regardless of your symptoms or how you respond to medication, you have to learn coping skills to change your life and manage your disorders. While medications are helpful for many disorders, other strategies are also needed, which is why counseling or therapy can help.

## Coping with People Who Pressure You to Stop Taking Medication

Since other people may suggest that you stop taking your medications, it helps to think ahead and plan how to handle this situation if it arises. You should think about this the same way you think about heart medication. If another person told you to get off your heart medication, would you stop it? Of course not! The same holds true for medication used for an addiction and/or a psychiatric illness. Tell people straight out that you need the medication, question why they would want you to stop a medication used to treat a serious disorder, or tell them that you don't appreciate their poor advice.

Some people believe they have to "white knuckle" it, that no matter how severe their symptoms, they should cope without medication. We have seen people suffer needlessly because they felt that they should not take medication. The reality is that some people cannot recover from an addiction or psychiatric disorder unless they are on medications. Remind yourself what can happen if you stop taking medication and the benefits you have experienced. Ask your sponsor or treatment team for other ideas or ways to cope with pressures from others to stop taking your medications. Ask other people in your program how they dealt with this pressure.

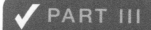

**PART III**

# Relapse Prevention, Progress Measurement, and Co-occurring Psychiatric Disorders

## CHAPTER 16

# Relapse Prevention
## *Reducing the Risk of Relapse*

## Goals

- To understand the difference between a lapse and relapse
- To learn about relapse prevention strategies
- To learn to identify and manage relapse warning signs and high-risk factors

## Lapse and Relapse

A *lapse* refers to an initial episode of substance use following a period of abstinence. A lapse may or may not lead to more substance use. You always run the risk that a lapse will turn into a *relapse*, in which you continue to use alcohol or other drugs.

A lapse or relapse is the last link in a chain of decisions. Before you pick up that first drink, cigarette, or other drug, you will make decisions that are "set-ups" for relapse. Going to a bar to drink soda 2 weeks after quitting alcohol is a relapse set-up. Hanging out with friends who snort cocaine or smoke marijuana and trying to abstain while they get high is a relapse set-up. This is why it's important to be aware of the seemingly irrelevant decisions that you usually make before your relapse. For example, Rick had abstained from alcohol for more than 7 months when he met someone at a bar to discuss a potential job. Although he had no intention of drinking when this arrangement was made, once he was in the bar, Rick found it impossible to resist his desires to drink. Amber stopped using heroin and was doing well in recovery. Following dental surgery, she took opioids for pain and got addicted again. Amber never told her counselor or Narcotics Anonymous (NA) sponsor about her dental surgery. Nor did she tell the dental surgeon about her history of opioid addiction. Both Rick and Amber made decisions that set them up for relapse.

## Response to a Lapse or Relapse

How you respond to an initial lapse has a big impact on whether or not you have a full-blown relapse. If you see yourself as a failure and say, "I'm not capable of stopping" or "I just can't control myself," you are likely to continue using. If you view your lapse as a mistake and an opportunity to strengthen your resolve, you can learn from it. Even if you end up having a full-blown relapse, you can learn by reviewing what led up to it, where, and how it happened.

## Relapse Prevention

Relapse prevention (RP) refers strategies and skills that you use to avoid substance use, modify your lifestyle, and reduce stress so that you lower your risk of relapse. Effective RP requires you to be motivated to change and to develop confidence in your ability to handle stressful situations.

RP involves thinking ahead and anticipating the problems or situations that could lead you back to alcohol, tobacco, or other drug use if you fail to use coping strategies. By identifying these potential problems (also referred to as "high-risk" situations) ahead of time, you can plan ways of coping with the problems without substance use. It's much better to have a plan for coping with a relapse and not need it than to need a plan and not have one. This is similar to the rationale for a fire drill: it's better to know what to do in case of a fire than to be caught off guard. RP prepares you ahead of time for what could happen.

*Relapse management* prepares you to handle actual lapses or relapses so that you can minimize the damage. You have to learn to act quickly and catch your mistakes before the situation worsens. Relapse management strategies are discussed in Chapter 17.

Learning to live a balanced life is an important issue in lowering your relapse risk. Chapter 18 focuses on strategies for *balanced living*. The better you can satisfy your needs, the less likely you are to want alcohol or other drugs.

## Warning Signs of Relapse

Before you lapse or relapse, you are likely to experience obvious and subtle warning signs that you are headed back toward substance use (Figure 16.1). These warning signs may show up in your attitudes and thoughts as well as in your behaviors and decisions.

As stated earlier, you may make decisions that initially seem to have little to do with a lapse or relapse but which, upon closer examination, are seen to be closely connected with it. For example, after being alcohol-free for 5 months, Andrew began to golf again with his former drinking buddies. By the third weekend of golf with these friends, his thoughts about having "a few drinks" had increased significantly, and Andrew told himself, "I can't fit in unless I drink with the guys." So, he drank again.

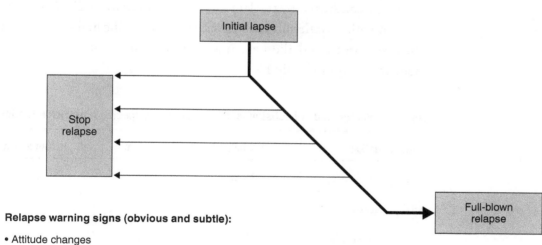

Relapse warning signs (obvious and subtle):

• Attitude changes

• Thought changes

• Mood changes

• Behavior changes

**Figure 16.1**

The relapse process.

Andrew also failed to share with his therapist when he initially thought that he had to drink to fit in with his golfing friends.

Complete Worksheet 16.1: Relapse Warning Signs, later in this chapter, to identify your relapse warning signs and strategies for coping with them. Keep in mind that the time between the emergence of relapse warning signs and actual substance use varies from person to person. The earlier you see the warning signs, the easier it will be to stop yourself before you pick up the first drink, cigarette, or other drug. Even if you have never relapsed, you will learn about relapse warning signs by the time you complete this chapter.

## High-Risk Situations

High-risk situations are those in which your vulnerability to using substances is moderate to high. High-risk situations are more likely to lead to relapse if you deny or minimize their existence or don't develop effective coping strategies when confronted with them. Leading an imbalanced lifestyle is likely to put you in high-risk situations. You might feel that you need to use substances to cope with upset feelings or a particular problem.

In a study conducted by the late Dr. G. Alan Marlatt, individuals with alcohol, nicotine, or heroin problems identified specific high-risk situations. These situations and the percentages of substance users who identified them are shown in Table 16.1.

**Table 16.1 Percentages of substance users identifying specific high-risk situations**

| Relapse situation | Alcoholics | Smokers | Heroin addicts |
|---|---|---|---|
| Negative emotions | 38% | 37% | 19% |
| Social pressures | 18% | 32% | 36% |
| Interpersonal conflict | 18% | 15% | 14% |
| Positive emotions | 3% | 9% | 15% |
| Urges, temptations | 11% | 5% | 5% |
| Other | 12% | 2% | 11% |

Complete Worksheet 16.2: High-Risk Situations. This will help you identify your potential relapse risks and develop positive coping strategies. It is important to think and plan ahead so that you are prepared to handle high-risk situations and will not be taken by surprise.

## Homework

- ✎ Complete Worksheet 16.1: Relapse Warning Signs.
- ✎ Complete Worksheet 16.2: High-Risk Situations.

**Worksheet 16.1**
**Relapse Warning Signs**

**Instructions:** In the left column, list the attitudes, thoughts, and behaviors that are warning signs for you of potential relapse. In the right column, write strategies for coping with each of these situations.

| Relapse warning signs | Coping strategies |
| --- | --- |
| _____ | _____ |
| _____ | _____ |
| _____ | _____ |
| _____ | _____ |
| _____ | _____ |
| _____ | _____ |
| _____ | _____ |
| _____ | _____ |
| _____ | _____ |
| _____ | _____ |
| _____ | _____ |
| _____ | _____ |
| _____ | _____ |
| _____ | _____ |
| _____ | _____ |
| _____ | _____ |
| _____ | _____ |
| _____ | _____ |

**Instructions:** List three of your high-risk situations below. For each high-risk situation, list positive coping strategies.

| High-risk situation 1 | Coping strategies |
| --- | --- |
| | |
| | |
| | |
| | |
| | |
| | |
| | |

| High-risk situation 2 | Coping strategies |
| --- | --- |
| | |
| | |
| | |
| | |
| | |
| | |
| | |

| High-risk situation 3 | Coping strategies |
| --- | --- |
| | |
| | |
| | |
| | |
| | |
| | |
| | |

## CHAPTER 17

# Relapse Management
## What to Do If You Lapse or Relapse

## Goals

- To determine and evaluate the reasons for your lapse or relapse
- To analyze the warning signs
- To learn the steps you should take when facing a lapse crisis
- For opioid-addicted individuals, to protect yourself from drug overdoses

## Learning from Your Past Mistakes

If you have a lapse or relapse, use it as a learning experience to help strengthen your recovery. Try to figure out your warning signs and the factors that led to your lapse or relapse. Use it as a motivator to change and to do things differently in your recovery. Complete Worksheet 17.1: Lapse and Relapse, later in this chapter, to help you evaluate what led to your first drink, cigarette, or use of another drug after having quit. If you have had more than one lapse or relapse, you can complete the worksheet based on several previous experiences. Then you can determine if there are any patterns to your return to substance use.

You should always inform your therapist or counselor if you have a lapse or relapse so that you can work together to figure out what caused it and how you can get back on track. Such open discussions will help you in the long run, even if you feel guilty or shameful about your lapse or relapse.

Your therapist is there to help you, not to judge you for any mistakes that you make.

## Identifying Your Relapse Chain

One helpful way of learning from your mistakes is to complete Worksheet 17.2: Relapse Chain, at the end of this chapter. This process involves a more detailed analysis in which you trace your lapse or relapse back to find warning signs that, in retrospect, you think were involved in your relapse process. Each warning sign, represented by one link in the relapse chain, involves a specific thought, feeling, or action that you believe was ultimately connected to your decision to use substances again. Complete Worksheet 17.2 after reading this chapter.

## Reactions to a Lapse or Relapse

The thoughts and feelings you experience following a lapse play a major role in whether or not you continue to use and move toward a full-blown relapse. Following your initial use of alcohol, tobacco, or other drugs, if you tell yourself, "I'm a failure, I can't do this, I'll never get it together," or "Since I can't stop myself from going back to using, I might as well continue," you are at high risk for a relapse because you'll be tempted to give up. If, after a lapse, you feel excited, happy, good, euphoric, mellow, or even relieved, you may easily ask yourself, "If substances make me feel this good, why not continue to use?" On the other hand, you may feel guilty, shameful, angry at yourself, or disappointed in yourself, only to use these emotions as motivators for continued substance use. Usually, the more negative your initial reaction to a lapse, the more likely you are to say, "The hell with it," and continue using.

Similarly, your thoughts and feelings about a relapse have an impact on whether or not you take action to stop the relapse and get back on the recovery track. If you see yourself as a failure or feel guilty and shameful, you may hesitate to ask a therapist, friend, or family member for help and support.

## Reactions of Family or Concerned Significant Others

Your family or others close to you may react negatively to your return to using substances, especially if you were addicted or your substance use had caused serious problems for you or your family. Some people may be supportive and understanding, but others may become upset and angry with you. When Franco relapsed, his family helped him stop it quickly by pointing out their observations and encouraging him to get back on track by increasing the frequency of his counseling sessions and attending more Narcotics Anonymous (NA) meetings. Since they attended some counseling sessions with Franco and also attended a family support program, they knew this was the most helpful approach to take with him rather than expressing anger and confronting him in a judgmental manner. On the other hand, Lisa's family was livid when she relapsed. This came after her fifth rehabilitation program. Prior to Lisa's relapse, her parents reached the point where they felt there was hope for her recovery. After this relapse, her dad told her he was done watching her kill herself and that it was up to Lisa to decide if she wanted to get her life together. Although her father's disappointment and pain are understandable, lashing out at his daughter was not helpful. Lisa felt awful and was ashamed because she had such a hard time sustaining her recovery. She worried that her parents would detach from her at a time when she believed their support is needed. When families react in a negative or judgmental way, or make threats, they are often doing this out of their love and fear for their family member because they hate to see them using drugs again. This is one of the reasons that involvement in some of your counseling sessions and/or attending family support programs can be vital for the health of your family.

## Steps to Take in a Lapse Crisis

The late Dr. G. Alan Marlatt outlined the following steps to reduce the damage of a lapse:

- *Stop, look, and listen.* Figure out what has caused you to lapse. Get out of high-risk situations immediately if there is a threat that your lapse will lead to a full-blown relapse.

- *Face your problems.* Deal with problems and crises immediately so that things don't build up to the point where you feel tempted to continue using alcohol or drugs.
- *Renew your commitment.* Remind yourself of your goals and of how important it is not to use alcohol or other drugs if you are to reach your goals.
- *Use your support network.* Ask family, friends, or others in recovery for help and support if needed.
- *Learn from your mistakes.* See what valuable lessons you can learn from your lapse. Think about ways to use this experience to help you in the future.

## If You Have an Opioid Use Disorder

Given the increase in rates of drug overdoses caused by heroin, fentanyl, and other opioids (sometimes mixed with other drugs), if you have an opioid use disorder make sure you get a Narcan kit so that an opioid drug overdose can be reversed by another person (friend, family member, or first responder). Ask you family or concerned significant other to learn how to administer this in case you overdose. This should be seen as a safety precaution, not as an endorsement to use drugs. Illicit drugs are sometimes more potent than expected or contain other drugs that increase the risk of overdose (such as fentanyl mixed with heroin or cocaine) without the user's knowledge.

## Homework

✎ Complete Worksheet 17.1: Lapse and Relapse.
✎ Complete Worksheet 17.2: Relapse Chain.

**Worksheet 17.1**
**Lapse and Relapse**

**Instructions:** Answer the following questions to help you figure out what led to your first drink, cigarette, or other drug use after having quit.

1. Describe the main reason you took the first drink, cigarette, or other drug.

   _____

   _____

   _____

   _____

2. Describe your inner thoughts and feelings that triggered your need or desire for the first drink, cigarette, or other drug.

   _____

   _____

   _____

   _____

3. Describe any external circumstances that triggered your need or desire for the first drink, cigarette, or other drug.

   _____

   _____

   _____

   _____

4. Describe the first decision you made that started the lapse or relapse process.

   _____

   _____

   _____

   _____

## Worksheet 17.2
## Relapse Chain

**Instructions:** The last link in the relapse chain represents your use of alcohol, tobacco, or other drugs. Each preceding link represents a specific relapse warning sign. Identify as many warning signs as you can. Then state how much time elapsed between the earliest warning sign and the first time you used a substance again. Also, state how you felt about using substances again and how your family (or other significant people in your life) felt.

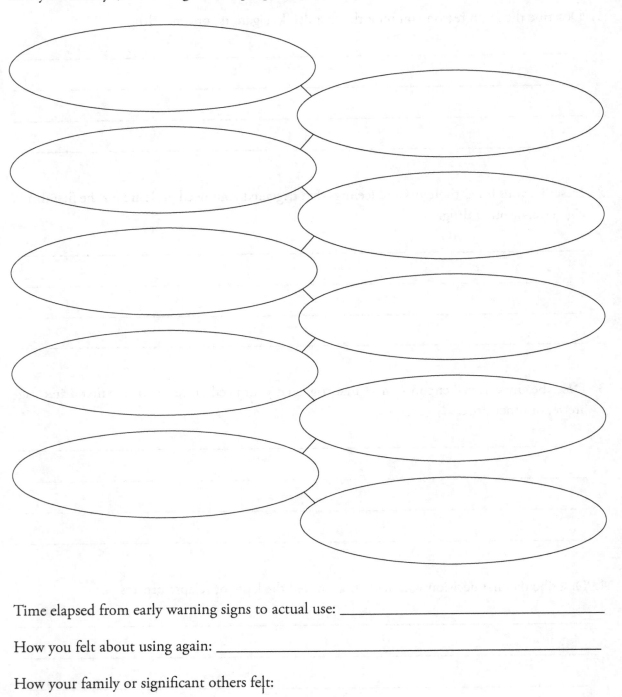

Time elapsed from early warning signs to actual use: _____

How you felt about using again: _____

How your family or significant others felt: _____

_____

# CHAPTER 18 ▶ Strategies for Balanced Living

## Goals

- To understand the benefits of living a balanced lifestyle
- To determine the overall balance of your life
- To learn how to keep a daily inventory to catch problems and relapse warning signs early
- To develop a weekly schedule of activities to add structure to your life
- To create a list of pleasant activities

## The Importance of Balance

*Balance* refers to the ability to reasonably manage the different aspects of your life. Balanced living is not only healthy but also serves as a protection against relapse. Balance can lead to happiness and give you an opportunity for personal growth. Although some areas of life may get temporarily out of balance due to demands of work or family, the goal is to strive for a balance that works for you and that can accommodate periods of imbalance.

Everyone has a number of responsibilities in life or things that "should" be done. Everyone has "wants" or individual needs and interests that are important, too. Balance implies making sure that some of your "wants" get taken care of so that all your energy isn't directed toward your obligations. If your "shoulds" (obligations) greatly outnumber your "wants" (desires), your life is out of balance. One way to find this out is to list your "wants" and "shoulds" on opposite sides of the Teeter-Totter Balance Test (see Worksheet 18.1, later in this chapter).

## Targeting Areas of Imbalance to Change

One helpful way to view the concept of balance is to examine your life from each of the following major perspectives to determine any areas of serious imbalance:

- physical,
- mental or emotional,
- intellectual,
- creative or artistic,
- family,
- personal relationships,
- spiritual,
- work or school, and
- financial.

Your particular needs in each area will depend on your personality, interests, and desire to change. Complete Worksheet 18.2: Lifestyle Balance, later in this chapter, to help you determine how balanced your life is overall. If a particular area is too much out of balance, think about steps you can take to change it.

## Daily Inventory or Review

Another approach to catching problems and relapse warning signs early is to take a few minutes at the end of each day to complete a review of your day. Ask yourself a few questions:

- Did any problems occur today that need my immediate attention?
- Did anything happen today that changed my desire or motivation to stay off alcohol, tobacco, or other drugs?
- Did I experience strong cravings or persistent thoughts of using today that are still with me?
- Did I notice any relapse indicators or warning signs today?

If you respond "Yes" to any of these questions, the next step is to develop a plan to deal with your relapse potential.

## Weekly Schedule

Developing a weekly schedule of activities is one way to add structure to your life. Your schedule will also give you an overview of the different things you are spending your time on, so you have an idea of the areas that need less or more attention. A weekly schedule, if reasonably balanced, can reduce the likelihood of your feeling bored or depressed. Plus, it will help you see some of the areas you are neglecting. For example, in reviewing several of his weekly schedules, it became clear to Dan that his schedule was so full of work-related activities that he left little time to spend with his kids or engage in regular exercise.

You can complete Worksheet 18.3: Weekly Schedule, to help plan your week. You may photocopy the worksheet from this workbook or download multiple copies at the Treatments *ThatWork* web site at www.oup. com/us/ttw. Although planning is especially helpful in the early phases of recovery, don't feel like you have to fill up all of your time. Leave some unstructured time so there's room for spontaneity and relaxation.

## Pleasant Activities

Participating in pleasant activities is another strategy for reducing boredom and depression and increasing positive feelings. As easy as this sounds, it is difficult for many people who give up using alcohol or other drugs. You can use Worksheet 18.4: Pleasant Activities, to identify current pleasant activities. You can also use this worksheet to identify potential pleasant activities. This offers you the opportunity to think about new activities that you would like to try. For example, when Regina examined her list of activities, she discovered that most of her pleasant activities revolved around her husband and children. Over the years, she had given up several activities she enjoyed either alone or with female friends, using the excuse that she was too busy to do these things. Unfortunately, the result was that Regina felt frustrated, resentful, and deprived. To gain more balance between her needs and the needs of her family, Regina began to take time for herself. She took a class on Chinese cooking with a girlfriend and started to go out to see new movies on occasion. Although she loves her kids dearly, Regina found the company of other adults to be pleasant and much needed.

## Homework

- ✎ Complete Worksheet 18.1: Teeter-Totter Balance Test.
- ✎ Complete Worksheet 18.2: Lifestyle Balance.
- ✎ Take a few minutes at the end of each day to complete a daily inventory.
- ✎ Complete Worksheet 18.3: Weekly Schedule to help plan your week.
- ✎ Complete Worksheet 18.4: Pleasant Activities.

# Worksheet 18.1
## Teeter-Totter Balance Test

**Wants List**                    **Shoulds List**

_____        _____

_____        _____

_____        _____

_____        _____

_____        _____

_____        _____

_____        _____

**Worksheet 18.2**
**Lifestyle Balance**

**Instructions:** Answer the following questions to help you determine how balanced your life is currently. Then review your answers. Identify two out-of-balance areas that you want to change. Write a plan for change in each area.

1. **Physical:**

   Are you in good health? ___Yes ___No

   Do you exercise regularly? ___Yes ___No

   Do you follow a reasonable diet? ___Yes ___No

   Do you take good care of your appearance? ___Yes ___No

   Do you get sufficient rest and sleep? ___Yes ___No

   Do you get regular medical and dental check-ups? ___Yes ___No

   Do you have strategies to handle cravings to use substances? ___Yes ___No

2. **Mental/emotional:**

   Are you experiencing excessive stress? ___Yes ___No

   Do you worry too much? ___Yes ___No

   Do you have strategies to reduce mental stress? ___Yes ___No

   Are you able to express your feelings to others? ___Yes ___No

   Do you suffer from depression or anxiety? ___Yes ___No

3. **Intellectual:**

   Are you able to satisfy your intellectual needs? ___Yes ___No

   Do you have enough interests to satisfy your curiosity? ___Yes ___No

4. **Creative/artistic:**

   Do you regularly participate in creative or artistic interests? ___Yes ___No

   Do you have talents or abilities that are not being used as much as you would like? ___Yes ___No

### 5. Family:

| | | |
|---|---|---|
| Are you satisfied with your family relationships? | ___Yes | ___No |
| Do you have any serious family problems that need to be addressed now? | ___Yes | ___No |
| Do you spend enough time with your family (including your children)? | ___Yes | ___No |
| Do you rely on your family for help and support? | ___Yes | ___No |

### 6. Personal relationships:

| | | |
|---|---|---|
| Are you satisfied with the quantity and quality of your personal relationships? | ___Yes | ___No |
| Is there enough love in your life? | ___Yes | ___No |
| Do you have friends you can depend on for help and support? | ___Yes | ___No |
| Are you able to express your ideas, needs, and feelings to others? | ___Yes | ___No |
| Are there any specific relationships in which you have serious problems? | ___Yes | ___No |

### 7. Spiritual:

| | | |
|---|---|---|
| Do you pay enough attention to your "inner" spiritual life? | ___Yes | ___No |
| Do you need to engage more in formal religion? | ___Yes | ___No |
| Are you satisfied with your spirituality (as you define it)? | ___Yes | ___No |
| Do you feel a sense of inner peace? | ___Yes | ___No |

### 8. Work or school

| | | |
|---|---|---|
| Are you usually satisfied with your work or school situation? | ___Yes | ___No |
| Do you spend too much time or effort working? | ___Yes | ___No |
| Do you spend too little time or effort working? | ___Yes | ___No |

### 9. Financial:

| | | |
|---|---|---|
| Do you have sufficient income to meet your expenses? | ___Yes | ___No |
| Are you having serious financial problems (e.g., too much debt, no savings)? | ___Yes | ___No |
| Do you handle your money responsibilities with an eye to the future? | ___Yes | ___No |
| Does money play too big a role in your life? | ___Yes | ___No |

**Out-of-balance area:**

_____

**My change plan:**

_____

_____

_____

_____

**Out-of-balance area:**

_____

**My change plan:**

_____

_____

_____

# Worksheet 18.3
## Weekly Schedule

| | Sunday | Monday | Tuesday | Wednesday | Thursday | Friday | Saturday |
|---|---|---|---|---|---|---|---|
| 6:00 | | | | | | | |
| 7:00 | | | | | | | |
| 8:00 | | | | | | | |
| 9:00 | | | | | | | |
| 10:00 | | | | | | | |
| 11:00 | | | | | | | |
| 12:00 | | | | | | | |
| 1:00 | | | | | | | |
| 2:00 | | | | | | | |
| 3:00 | | | | | | | |
| 4:00 | | | | | | | |
| 5:00 | | | | | | | |
| 6:00 | | | | | | | |
| 7:00 | | | | | | | |
| 8:00 | | | | | | | |
| 9:00 | | | | | | | |
| 10:00 | | | | | | | |
| 11:00 | | | | | | | |

**Worksheet 18.4**
**Pleasant Activities**

**Instructions:** List current activities that you consider to be a pleasant part of your life. Then think of several new activities to try. These should be activities in which there is no or minimal pressure to use alcohol or other drugs.

**Current pleasant activities:**

_____

_____

_____

_____

_____

_____

**New pleasant activities:**

_____

_____

_____

_____

_____

_____

## Goals

- To learn to define and measure the progress you've made thus far
- To recognize that progress shows in many aspects of your life, just not substance use

## How to Define Progress

You can measure your progress by comparing your current status to the goals you set at the beginning of your change program (for example, see Worksheets 4.1 and 7.1). These goals may relate to your substance use; to any area of your life, such as physical, mental, or spiritual well-being, or your relationships with family or friends; or to any other problem or issue that you are working on changing.

Progress is improvement or positive movement toward your identified goals. Sometimes progress is significant and happens quickly. Other times progress is less significant and happens slowly. Try to avoid the trap of judging progress in absolute or "all or none" terms because you can be making progress even if you still have problems. For instance, Curtis has not reached his goal of sustained abstinence from cocaine and heroin. However, in the past year, he's used on fewer than 30 days, which is significantly better than his daily use during the previous year. Amanda identified the goal of "learning to cope with my anger and rage and express it appropriately." During the past 3 months, she's had only two minor episodes of lashing out at her husband and kids—much better than when she used to lash out a couple of times every week. Although Amanda has gained greater control over her feelings and behavior, she is still working on this problem.

## Ongoing Abstinence

For many people in recovery, ongoing abstinence from alcohol, drugs, or tobacco is the primary goal in the early phases of recovery. If you've been able to achieve and maintain total abstinence, that is great! Keep doing what helps you stay substance-free. If you've been unable to maintain total abstinence, try to figure out the problems that get in your way and learn from your experiences with relapse. It is not unusual for some people to make several tries at abstinence before being able to maintain it continuously. If you cannot sustain abstinence from an opioid, alcohol, or tobacco use disorder with counseling and/or mutual support programs, consider medications, as we discussed in Chapter 15 of this workbook. Medications can reduce substance cravings and regulate your brain chemistry, making it easier for you to focus on personal or lifestyle changes.

## Reduction of Substance Use

Another way of measuring progress is to see if you've reduced the amount and frequency of substance use (harm reduction). If you have been unable to achieve total abstinence but you are using smaller quantities and less often, this is a step in the right direction. You are making progress. Although total abstinence is best if you have an alcohol or drug use disorder, reduction of use with less severe substance use problems can be a reasonable goal, but only if you don't have significant medical, psychiatric, or other problems caused or worsened by substance use. It is also best not to use any illicit drugs.

## Decrease in Harmful Effects of Substances

Another way of measuring progress is to look at the effects of your substance use. If you are having fewer or less severe problems resulting from substance use, then you are headed in the right direction. For example, Melanie has managed to reduce her substance use by about 80%. She recognizes that she still needs help and is working toward total abstinence. Melanie has significantly reduced her alcohol use and completely stopped her marijuana use, resulting in fewer disagreements with her husband, no missed work due to hangovers, and no spending money that should go toward bills. She no longer feels hopeless. Seeing her life improve has given Melanie an incentive to continue working hard at achieving and maintaining abstinence from alcohol and marijuana.

## Improvement in Functioning and Quality of Life

Usually, if you stop or cut down on your substance use, you will experience improvement in the quality of your life. Jenny, for example, has more stamina when she climbs the stairs at work since she quit smoking. Destiny is able to function as a responsible mother now that she stays off marijuana. Anthony has begun to save for his own apartment since he quit alcohol and other drugs. Huang has gained 25 pounds and is close to his ideal body weight since quitting cocaine. The ways of measuring specific progress in the quality of your health and life are endless. Even small or modest changes show you are progressing in your recovery.

## Reduction of Obsessions and Cravings

You are making progress when your desires, obsessions, or cravings for alcohol, tobacco, or other drugs are less intense, less frequent, or less bothersome. For some, it is a blessing to lose the obsession about using alcohol or other drugs. Successfully managing and living with your cravings is another indication that you are doing better. For example, Phil used to feel tortured by his intense desires to use heroin in the early weeks of recovery. What helps him now is taking the medication buprenorphine and sharing his cravings with peers in a mutual support group. Wendy still sometimes thinks about drinking but says her cravings are less intense now. She reminds herself "this (craving) too shall pass" and coaches herself into "putting off drinking until the next day or so." By that time, Wendy's alcohol craving usually is gone or is mild.

## Increased Confidence in Your Ability to Cope

Feeling more confident in your ability to cope with cravings, pressures to use, or other problems is another sign of progress. Except in cases of false confidence or overconfidence, the more confidence you have in your ability to successfully cope with high-risk situations, the more likely you are to handle these situations without using. For example, in the past, Jose started using again after giving in to pressure to party with friends he used to get high with. Since he has now resisted numerous attempts to drink or smoke pot, Jose believes he has the ability to sustain his recovery regardless of what people try to get him to do.

## Increased Awareness of High-Risk Situations

Another sign of progress is increased awareness of your high-risk situations and an ability to face them rather than ignoring them or minimizing their potential to cause relapse. A greater awareness of your high-risk situations allows you to develop coping strategies. It also decreases the likelihood that you will set yourself up for relapse by putting yourself in situations in which you feel unable to resist the desire to use alcohol, tobacco, or other drugs. For example, Lauren accepts that, for the time being, she will not attend any music concerts because smelling pot taps into her desire to get high. Lauren knows that avoiding concerts is her best strategy at this time, but, later on, she may be able to attend concerts without worrying about getting high.

## Willingness to Discuss a Close Call, Lapse, or Relapse

Progress can also relate to changes in your attitude or in how you use this recovery program and work with a therapist. Even if you are struggling with using, if you are willing to talk about lapses or relapses, close calls, and other problems that you are experiencing, then you open the door for progress in your recovery. Learning to talk about yourself and to trust your therapist are good signs of progress; this helps your therapist better understand and work with you. For example, Jerry lied to his therapist after drinking several times. When he finally opened up and told the truth about his struggle, he felt better about himself and believes this will help his recovery. His therapist thanked him for sharing this and reinforced his desire to work with Jerry and to not judge him for any episodes of use. Jerry was relieved and realized he and his therapist really were a team working together on his recovery.

## Willingness to Change Your Recovery Plan

If your current recovery plan is not working, whether it's one you devised on your own or with the help of a therapist, then change your plan and your approach to recovery. You've no doubt heard the saying "If it ain't broke, don't fix it." The opposite is true if you aren't making progress in recovery: "If it's not working, change it." For example, Janine's therapist recommended that she come to clinic three days per week to attend treatment groups and individual therapy. Janine did not think she needed this and requested individual counseling every two weeks. Since she was unable to remain abstinent from drugs, Janine reluctantly agreed to attend a more intensive level of treatment. It turned out that this helped her put together a longer period of sustained recovery. Janine had the insight to realize that changing "her plan," being open-minded, and following the recommended plan of her therapist was in her best interests.

## Increase in Community Involvement

Although this may not be a goal for you, progress can also show in greater engagement in your community. This may involve participation in school, religious or civic groups or activities, volunteering for a community or mutual help organization that could use your talents and time, or being more active in important civic duties such as voting. For example, Don returned to regular church attendance after years of missing due to his drug problem. And he now votes in local, state, and national elections after not doing so for more than 20 years.

## Final Thoughts

Your willingness to become involved in a recovery program shows that you want to do something to manage your substance use problem. There are no guarantees, the work of recovery is not always easy, and progress is sometimes gradual. However, sticking with your recovery plan and changing it when it's not working can help you stop using substances and make positive changes in yourself. Keys to success include:

- using active coping skills to manage the challenges of recovery;
- setting goals and working toward them;
- sticking with your treatment until you complete it;
- actively participating in a mutual support program;
- taking medications if they are prescribed;
- not making private decisions to quit treatment or mutual support participation without discussing this with someone else; and
- learning from any mistakes you make.

Completing Worksheet 19.1: Putting It All Together: What You Have Learned and What You Will Continue to Do to Change, can help you to remember and continue using the skills you've learned during your recovery. Educating yourself and learning appropriate coping skills can help you learn to manage your alcohol or drug problem and improve your life.

## Homework

✎ Complete Worksheet 19.1: Putting It All Together: What You Have Learned and What You Will Continue to Do to Change.

## Worksheet 19.1

### Putting It All Together: What You Have Learned and What You Will Continue to Do to Change

1. Summarize what you have learned about yourself from completing this workbook and developing a change program with your therapist or counselor.

_____

_____

_____

_____

_____

_____

_____

_____

2. Summarize how you will continue to make positive changes in your life to help you stay alcohol- and drug-free.

_____

_____

_____

_____

_____

_____

_____

## CHAPTER 20

Managing a Co-occurring
Psychiatric Disorder

## Goals

- To learn about the different types of psychiatric disorders
- To learn about the causes of psychiatric disorders
- To assess your psychiatric symptoms, if applicable

## Introduction

The term "co-occurring disorders" refers to the presence of a psychiatric disorder (such as bipolar disorder) and a substance use disorder (SUD; such as alcohol use disorder). A psychiatric disorder increases the risk of a SUD and vice versa. Treating one disorder improves the outcomes in treating the other. Psychiatric medications can be both effective and appropriate in treating the psychiatric disorder in people with co-occurring disorders. And medication-assisted treatment (MAT) can treat effectively the SUD in people with co-occurring disorders. You need to think of recovery as something that goes beyond the disorders, which means working your recovery through rebuilding your value system and reclaiming your identity.

## What Is Mental Health?

Mental "health" implies the absence of a psychiatric (mental) disorder. It involves the ability to anticipate and solve problems, manage emotions, deal with frustrations and setbacks, set goals, maintain satisfying relationships, and function responsibly in society.

A person does not have either "mental health" or a "mental or psychiatric disorder." Rather, there are degrees of mental health and degrees of severity of psychiatric disorders. For example, even people who are psychologically healthy can feel anxious or depressed at times. On the other hand, people with psychiatric disorders may have problems in some areas of life and do well in other areas. For example, Matt has a depressive disorder, and Serena has an eating disorder. Both do well in school, yet other areas of their health and life are affected by their disorders, such as their relationships with their significant others and family members and their struggles with having a balanced lifestyle.

Factors that protect a person or reduce the risk of developing a psychiatric disorder include (1) strong bonds with family, community, school, or religious organization; (2) good coping skills to deal with emotions, problems, and social relationships; and (3) resiliency or ability to bounce back from difficulties.

## What Is a Psychiatric Disorder?

Almost one in four adults in the United States experiences a psychiatric disorder (also called a *mental illness*) at some point in their lives. Many people have more than one disorder. Many others also have a SUD in addition to their psychiatric disorder(s). Psychiatric disorders involve a combination of symptoms that cause suffering and interfere with your ability to function. Each disorder has symptoms that relate to

- Moods and emotional states (how you feel and your emotional experiences)
- Thinking (how you interpret the world or events)
- Behavior (how you act)
- Physical health (your body)

Psychiatric disorders include single-episode, recurrent-episode, and chronic or persistent types. You can experience a single episode of illness and then return to normal, or you may have several episodes over time. The length of each episode will vary, as will the amount of time between episodes. You may experience chronic or persistent symptoms over time, which require that you manage symptoms that never totally go away. For example, your mood may improve, your anxiety level may go down, or your psychotic symptoms may lessen, but these symptoms may not go away totally. If you learn to control and live with these symptoms, the quality of your life can improve. After reading this chapter, complete Worksheet 20.1: Assessing Your Psychiatric Symptoms, at the end of this chapter.

## Types of Psychiatric Disorders

### Mood Disorders

Mood disorders involve disturbances in mood along with physical and behavioral symptoms. The most common is *major depression*, which involves feeling sad or blue, a loss of or decrease in interest in life and pleasurable activities, difficulty concentrating, appetite or sleep problems, tiredness or low energy, feelings of guilt and worthlessness, and thoughts about whether or not life is worth living. These symptoms are present most of the time, nearly every day, for 2 weeks or longer.

Another form is *recurrent depression*. This involves three or more different episodes of major depression over time. Months or years may separate these episodes. About half of people with depression will have a recurrent course of this disorder. *Persistent depressive disorder* (previously called *dysthymia*) is a chronic form of depression and involves feeling depressed most days for at least 2 years with two or more of the symptoms of major depression.

*Mania* is the opposite of depression in that the mood is elevated or "high" instead of depressed. Energy and activity levels increase and the need for sleep decreases. People with mania are easily distracted and their thoughts may race. During a conversation, they may jump from topic to topic. Since their judgment is affected, they may do foolish things, go on spending sprees, put themselves in danger, or get involved in a lot of activities at once.

Some people switch back and forth between depression and mania, an illness called *bipolar disorder* or *manic-depressive illness*. Some even experience symptoms of both depression and mania at the same time, a condition called *bipolar disorder, mixed type*.

## Anxiety Disorders

Anxiety disorders involve worrying too much, feeling a sense of dread, or feeling anxious or fearful. These disorders usually include both physical and mental symptoms. Many people have more than one anxiety disorder as well as depression and/or a SUD.

A *specific phobia* is an irrational fear of a situation or object so strong that it causes distress and problems in your life. *Social phobia* involves fear of being looked at, criticized, or rejected by others, or acting in ways that will be embarrassing or humiliating. Some people have many social situations they are afraid of, while others fear only one or two situations. Common social phobias include dating, speaking, writing or eating in public, and taking tests. *Specific phobias* involve irrational fears of situations such as being in a closed space, being in a high place, traveling by bus or plane, or fears of objects such as bugs, snakes, blood, or needles. One type of phobia, called *agoraphobia*, often makes the person a prisoner at home due to the fear of leaving. Many people with this disorder also have panic attacks.

*Panic disorder* involves sudden panic attacks in which the person feels an intense and overwhelming feeling of terror. The person may worry about going crazy or dying or feel that things "don't seem real." He or she may feel dizzy or faint, shake or tremble, sweat, feel sick to the stomach, or experience hot or cold flashes, chest pain, or a racing heart.

*Generalized anxiety disorder* involves continuous, unrealistic, and excessive anxiety and worry about two or more areas of life. This anxiety and worry is accompanied by symptoms such as trembling, feeling shaky, feeling restless, shortness of breath, increased heart rate, feeling dizzy, nausea, hot flashes or chills, feeling hyper, feeling keyed up or on edge, having trouble concentrating or "going blank," and irritability.

## Obsessive-Compulsive Disorders

*Obsessive-compulsive disorder* involves repeating behaviors over and over, like hand washing; checking doors, windows, or the stove; or counting objects many times. The person with this disorder often believes bad things will happen if these rituals are not repeated a certain number of times. This disorder also involves the recurrence of obsessions or senseless and frightening thoughts, over and over again. These obsessions or intruding thoughts can relate to harming yourself or another, germs or contamination, doing something embarrassing or out of the ordinary, something "real bad" happening, your body, or sex. Other obsessive-compulsive disorders include hoarding disorder, trichotillomania (hair-pulling disorder), and body dysmorphic disorders.

## Trauma- and Stressor-Related Disorders

This group of disorders includes posttraumatic stress disorder (PTSD), which involves reexperiencing past traumatic events months or years later. These events may relate to physical or sexual assault, a natural disaster, or military combat. PTSD symptoms show up in bad dreams, intrusive thoughts, or upsetting memories and cause depression, anxiety, and severe distress.

Other disorders in this category include adjustment disorder and acute stress disorder.

## Psychotic Disorders

Disorders such as *schizophrenia* involve unusual experiences such as hearing, feeling, seeing, or smelling things that are not there and that others do not experience. People with this illness may hear voices inside their head or have strange beliefs such as "others are out to get me" or "others are trying to put thoughts in my mind." Some sufferers exhibit strange or unusual behaviors like talking to themselves in public or dressing in a bizarre manner. Low motivation and social isolation are also common. The person with a psychotic disorder may lack emotion, feel flat, feel strange, have mood swings, or feel disconnected from other people.

## Eating Disorders

These disorders include anorexia and bulimia. *Anorexia* is a disorder in which the person limits food intake and is significantly below normal body weight. *Bulimia* is a disorder in which the person eats in a binge pattern and then induces vomiting or diarrhea to avoid gaining weight. Both disorders are associated with serious medical problems and other psychiatric disorders such as depression.

### Personality Disorders

These disorders occur when long-standing personality traits, or usual ways of thinking about and dealing with life or relating to other people, cause considerable distress or difficulty. Some examples of personality traits that may cause serious problems include being impulsive and failing to plan ahead or acting before you think; avoiding situations in which you are faced with problems or conflicts with people; or being antisocial, overly controlling, passive, aggressive, self-centered, perfectionistic, or dependent. For example, Julie has a borderline disorder. During times of excessive stress, she sometimes gets drunk. She also gets into verbal spats with friends, often exaggerating her emotions and blaming others for her problems. Mike, who has antisocial disorder, has a long history of doing whatever he feels like doing without considering the impact of his decisions on himself or other people. He recently got ticked off at his boss and abruptly quit his job without having another one. Mike also expresses intense emotions to control others by making them afraid of him.

### Co-occurring Disorders

Many people have both a psychiatric disorder and a substance use disorder. Having a psychiatric illness increases your risk of a SUD. Likewise, having a SUD increases your risk of psychiatric illness. Alcohol and drugs can make your psychiatric symptoms worse or can cause new symptoms. Some people go to a psychiatric hospital after using drugs or alcohol and becoming depressed, manic, psychotic, violent, or suicidal.

## Causes of Psychiatric Disorders

There is no simple way to explain why a given person develops a psychiatric disorder. Many biological, psychological, and environmental factors cause these disorders.

### Biological Factors

Just as diabetes, hypertension, or other medical problems run in families, so do psychiatric disorders. Scientists believe that some people inherit a predisposition to develop a psychiatric disorder. There may be something in brain chemistry that puts a person at risk for developing a disorder—he or she may be "wired" differently than others. This difference—rooted in biology—shows up in personality traits and behaviors and in how you process information, solve problems, and deal with your emotions. Heredity stacks the deck against some people. Therefore, it is not your fault if you have a psychiatric disorder, but it is your responsibility to do something about it and get the help you need.

### Psychological Factors

How you think, your personality, and how you deal with problems or manage stress have an impact on psychiatric disorders. Some people have fewer coping skills or are more sensitive to stress, negative emotions, or inaccurate thinking than others. Some people have a greater need to take risks in order to feel excitement, which can lead to problems because rules and laws are broken and risks are taken that can have grave consequences.

### Environmental and Genetic Factors

Family, social, or environmental factors contribute to psychiatric illness. Examples include a chaotic home environment in which parents are not consistent with discipline, are not predictable, or are perfectionistic and too demanding. Growing up in a home with a parent who has mental illness can raise your risk of illness. We have recently made considerable progress in understanding the genetics of SUDs. Genetic influences interact with environmental factors. At this point in time, we have a long way to go before we can identify any specific genes involved in specific SUDs.

## Effects of Psychiatric Disorders

The effects of a psychiatric illness depend on the type of illness, the severity of symptoms, whether or not you have more than one disorder or a coexisting SUD, and your personal characteristics. Psychiatric disorders may cause or worsen problems with your physical health, relationships, ability to succeed at school or work, and self-esteem. They can cause suicidal thinking or behaviors. These disorders also create a burden for families.

## Homework

✎ Complete Worksheet 20.1: Assessing Your Psychiatric Symptoms.

**Worksheet 20.1**
**Assessing Your Psychiatric Symptoms**

---

Following is a brief list of symptoms of the most common psychiatric disorders. Put a check mark (✓) next to the symptoms or behaviors that you currently are experiencing or you are concerned about because of past experiences.

**Mood Symptoms**
- ☐ Depression or sadness that will not go away
- ☐ Seldom feel pleasure or joy in life
- ☐ Feel hopeless or helpless
- ☐ Low energy or low motivation (hard to get moving)
- ☐ Poor appetite (eat too much or too little)
- ☐ Poor sleep patterns (hard to fall or stay asleep, sleep too little or too much)
- ☐ Hard to concentrate or solve problems
- ☐ Mania (high moods)
- ☐ Mood swings (switch back and forth between depression and high moods)
- ☐ Racing thoughts that are hard to control (hard to stick with one topic)
- ☐ Get involved in too many projects at the same time
- ☐ Sleep very little or go days without sleep
- ☐ Go on spending sprees or make bad decisions with money
- ☐ Get involved in risky behaviors (substance use, driving too fast, sex with strangers)
- ☐ Suicidal thoughts, plans or attempt

**Anxiety Symptoms**
- ☐ Severe anxiety or worry
- ☐ Avoiding situations that cause anxiety
- ☐ Panic attacks (racing heart, fears, worry about going crazy or dying)
- ☐ Strong fears or phobias (leaving home, flying, closed spaces, heights, animals)
- ☐ Bad memories, feeling or intrusive thoughts about physical/sexual abuse
- ☐ Obsessive thoughts (you repeat thoughts that intrude your mind)
- ☐ Compulsions (you repeat behaviors such as checking, counting, or washing)

**Psychotic Symptoms**
- ☐ Unusual experiences (you hear, feel, see, or smell things others do not)
- ☐ Unusual beliefs or delusions (being special, watched by others, or paranoid)
- ☐ Thinking difficulty (confused, cannot concentrate, have strange thoughts)
- ☐ Behavior changes (you stop eating or act very strangely)
- ☐ Mood changes (you feel strange, flat, or have mood swings)
- ☐ Negative symptoms (low motivation, social isolation, decreased thoughts)

**Eating Symptoms**
- ☐ Making yourself vomit after eating
- ☐ Too much dieting
- ☐ Eating too little due to fear of gaining weight or becoming fat

☐ Constant worry about weight gain or appearance
☐ Frequent use of diuretics or enemas

## Attention Deficit Symptoms

☐ Hard to pay attention, listen, or finish things (at home, school, work)
☐ Hard to focus on a task for very long
☐ Hard to get organized (at home, work, or school)
☐ Feeling hyper, restless, on edge, like your "motor" is always running
☐ Hard to sit still for very long
☐ Get frustrated very easily, even with small things
☐ Do things impulsively by acting before thinking of consequences

## Behavioral Symptoms and Relationship Problems

☐ Self-harm (cutting or burning self, overdosing on pills, etc.)
☐ Bad temper problem
☐ Bully, threaten, or intimidate other people
☐ Used a weapon to hurt or threaten others (bat, brick, knife, glass, gun)
☐ Violence toward people (hit, slap, push, punch, kick)
☐ Serious problems with spouse, parent, or other family member
☐ Serious problems in relationships
☐ Lying, conning, or deceiving others
☐ Trouble at work (missing days, late, getting fired, can't find or hold job)
☐ Trouble with school (skipping, bad grades, don't do work, kicked out/quit)
☐ Trouble with the law (arrested, did time in jail, on probation or parole)

## Other Symptoms (write in)

_____

_____

1. List below your psychiatric disorder(s). If you do not know your diagnosis, ask your doctor or therapist.

_____

_____

2. Describe how your life has been affected by your psychiatric disorder(s).

_____

_____

3. Describe what you hope to get out of treatment for your psychiatric disorders.

_____

_____

# Helpful Resources

These resources provide a rich array of educational materials, recovery tools, and treatment and recovery resources for practitioners, individuals with substance-related disorders, and families or significant others who are affected by a loved one's substance problems. Many of these websites include free PDF files that you can save on your computer or print. For practitioners, many treatment manuals, research papers, and treatment protocols are available that address assessment and treatment of substance-related disorders. For individuals and families, many articles, guides, and information sheets on substances and treatment and recovery from substance-related problems are available. Some resources, such as many of the mutual support programs, include online meetings or chat rooms. Others provide phone numbers to call for information about treatment services or for help and support for a family member or friend with a substance use disorder or for yourself. You can also get information and referral information from local and state organizations that focus on helping individuals or families affected by substance-related problem. You may need to insert http:// before the website addresses.

## US Government National Organizations

1. **National Institute on Alcohol Abuse and Alcoholism (NIAAA)** provides information on alcohol, alcohol-related problems, treatment, and recovery. www.niaaa.nih.gov

2. **National Institute on Drug Abuse (NIDA)** provides information on all types of drugs, drug-related problems, treatment, and recovery. Includes information to help young kids and teens learn about how drugs affect the brain and behavior. www.nida.nih.gov

3. **Substance Abuse and Mental Health Services Administration (SAMHSA)** offers free, confidential help lines every day of the year, 24/7, to provide information, referral, and/or help for (a) individuals or families affected by a substance use disorder or a mental health disorder (1-800-662-4357); (b) individuals in distress who are suicidal

(1-800-273-8255); and (c) individuals in distress who need crisis help due to a disaster (1-800-985-5990). www.samhsa.gov

## Mutual Support Programs for Alcohol or Drug Problems

1. **Alcoholics Anonymous (AA)** is a mutual support program for anyone with an alcohol problem who wants to stop drinking. AA has "tools" such as recovery meetings, sponsorship, recovery literature, the 12-step program, and many other resources. www.aa.org; *AA Online Chat* meetings are also available at www.aa-alive.net
2. **Alcoholics Victorious** is a program for individuals with alcohol or drug problems that uses the 12-steps of AA and readings from the Bible to promote recovery, with a focus on using Jesus as the "Higher Power." www.alcoholicsvictorious.org
3. **Narcotics Anonymous (NA)** is a mutual support program for individuals with any type of drug problem. It offers "tools" such as recovery meetings, sponsorship, recovery literature, the 12-step program, and other resources. www.na.org; *NA Online Chat* meetings are also available at www.nachatroom.org
4. **SMART Recovery (Self-Management and Recovery Training)** is a program for recovery from all types of addiction, including alcohol and drug addictions. It offers a 4-point program, meetings in person or online, chat rooms, and recovery literature. www.smartrecovery.org
5. **Women for Sobriety** is a program that helps women find their individual path to recovery through discovery of self gained by sharing experiences, hopes, and encouragement with other women in similar circumstances. Online meetings available and meeting finder. womenforsobriety.org/about

## Family Resources

1. **Al-Anon** is a mutual support program for friends and families of individuals with alcohol problems. Al-Anon offers group meetings (in-person, by phone, online, international) where friends and family members share their experiences and learn ways to cope with the effects of the alcohol problem on themselves. al-anon.org; *Al-Anon Online Chat* meetings are available on www.stepchat.com/alanon.htm

2. **Alateen** is a program for teens whose lives have been affected by someone else's drinking. Like Al-Anon, Alateen provides group meetings where members share experiences and learn the principles of the Al-Anon program. al-anon.org/newcomers/teen-corner-alateen

3. **Community Reinforcement Approach and Family Training (CRAFT)** is an approach to help families and significant others deal with a substance use problem in the family. It provides guidance on how to engage the member with the substance problem in treatment. It also helps the family deal with their own reactions to a loved one and engage in their own recovery. www.robertjmeyersphd.com/craft

4. **Dr. Dennis C. Daley's website** includes treatment manuals for professionals and recovery materials for individuals and family members covering substance use disorders, psychiatric disorders, and co-occurring disorders (both disorders combined). www.drdenniscdaley.com

5. **Faces and Voices of Recovery** is an advocacy organization that provides information and support for families and those with a substance use disorder. www.facesandvoicesofrecovery.org

6. **Facing Addiction** is an advocacy organization dedicated to finding solutions to the addiction crisis. They aim to build a national constituency, increase access to treatment, translate scientific innovation into services, advocate for governments to implement evidence-based policies, and share the proof of long-term recovery. www.facingaddiction.org

7. **Family Resource Center** website has various resources for families to understand and address a child's substance use. The resources can be filtered by the intended user; for example, parents of young adolescents, older teens, adult children, or teachers/community support personnel. www.familyresourcectr.org/category/community

8. **Families Anonymous** is for the families and friends who have known a feeling of desperation concerning the destructive behavior of someone very near to them, whether caused by drugs, alcohol, or related behavioral problems. *Meetings Without Walls* are online meetings. www.familiesanonymous.org

9. **Nar-Anon** is a 12-step mutual support program adopted from Narcotics Anonymous. This program offers group meetings and recovery tools for families affected by any type of drug problem. www.nar-anon.org/

10. **National Association of Children of Alcoholics** offers a rich array of information and resources on substance use problems and recovery

for families and children of all ages, and for professionals. You can access written and video materials, webinars, research reports, and stories of recovery of family members affected by a loved one's substance use disorder. www.nacoa.org

11. **Partnership for Drug-Free Kids** is a nonprofit organization that aims to help families struggling with their child's substance use. They provide information, support, and guidance to families, in addition to advocating for greater understanding and more effective programs to treat addiction. They offer a helpline that helps families connect with experts. www.drugfree.org

12. **SAMSHA—20 Minute Guide** is a free online resource for parents and partners about how they can help change their children's substance use. https://the20minuteguide.com

# Suggested Readings

Information in this workbook comes from a variety of sources. This includes books, articles, and studies on treatment of substance use disorders; reports by the US government; treatment manuals published by the National Institute on Drug Abuse; surveys of recovery or involvement in mutual support programs; and other recovery literature. We also incorporate knowledge gained from our decades of clinical experience working with thousands of individuals with all types of alcohol and drug problems and with families and concerned significant others affected by a loved one's problems, developing clinical treatment programs, writing treatment manuals, and participating in clinical research. We also include information from the research and clinical writings of the late Dr. G. Alan Marlatt who co-authored the first two editions of this workbook.

Alcoholics Anonymous World Service. (2001). *Alcoholics Anonymous*, 4th ed. New York: Author.

Alcoholics Anonymous World Service. (2014). *Alcoholics Anonymous 2013 membership survey*. New York: Author.

American Psychiatric Association. (2013). Substance-related and addictive disorders. In *Diagnostic and Statistical Manual of Mental Disorders* (DSM-5; 5th ed., pp. 481–590). Washington, DC: Author, 481–590.

American Society of Addiction Medicine. (2013). *The ASAM criteria: Treatment criteria for addictive, substance-related, and co-occurring conditions*, 3rd ed. David Mee-Lee (Ed.). Chevy Chase, MD.

Amin, P., & Douaihy, A. (2018). Substance use disorders in people living with HIV. *Nursing Clinics of North America, 53*, 57–65.

Center for Substance Abuse Treatment (CSAT). (2004). *Substance abuse treatment and family therapy. Treatment improvement protocol series*, TIP 39. Rockville, MD: SAMSHA.

Center for Substance Abuse Treatment (CSAT). (2005). *Substance abuse treatment for persons with co-occurring disorders*, TIP 42. Rockville, MD: SAMHSA.

Centers for Disease Control and Prevention (CDCP). (2017). Tobacco-related mortality. www.cdc.gov/tobacco/data_statistics/fact_sheets/fast_facts/. Accessed July 6, 2018.

Centers for Disease Control and Prevention (CDCP). (2018). Fact sheets on excessive alcohol use, binge drinking, underage drinking, and alcohol use and health. www.cdc.gov/alcohol/factsheets. Accessed July 6, 2018.

Cloninger, C. R. (2005). Genetics of substance abuse. In M. Galanter & H. D. Kleber (Eds.), *Textbook of substance abuse* (3rd ed., pp. 73–80). Washington, DC: American Psychiatric Publishing.

Daley, D. C. (2011). *Relapse prevention workbook*. Murrysville, PA: Daley Publications.

Daley, D. C. (2012). *Coping with feelings and moods: Recovery strategies for emotional health*. Murrysville, PA: Daley Publications.

Daley, D. C., Douaihy, A. D., Weiss, R. D., & Mercer, D. E. (2014). Group therapies. In R. K. Ries, D. A. Fiellin, S. C. Miller, & R. Saitz (Eds.), *The ASAM principles of addiction medicine* (5th ed., pp. 845–857). New York: Wolters Kluwer.

Daley, D. C., & Douaihy, A. D. (2006). *Addiction and mood disorders*. New York: Oxford University Press.

Daley, D. C., & Douaihy, A. D. (2014). *Recovery from co-occurring disorders: Staying sober and managing your psychiatric illness*. Murrysville, PA: Daley Publications.

Daley, D. C., & Douaihy, A. D. (2015). *Relapse prevention counseling: Clinical strategies to guide addiction recovery and reduce relapse*. Eau Claire, WI: PESI Publishing and Media.

Daley, D. C., & Miller, J. (2001). *Addiction in your family: Helping yourself and your loved ones*. Holmes Beach, FL: Learning Publications.

Daley, D. C., Smith, E., Balogh, D., & Toscolan, I. J. (2018). Forgotten but not gone: Impact of opioid and other substance use disorders on families and children. *Commonwealth, 20*(2–3), 93–121.

Daley, D. C., & Thase, M. E. (2004). *Dual disorders recovery counseling: Integrated treatment for substance use and mental health disorders*, 3rd ed. Independence, MO: Independence Press.

Daley, D. C., & Zuckoff, A. (1999). *Improving treatment compliance: Counseling and systems strategies for substance use and dual disorders*. Center City, MN: Hazelden.

Donovan, D. M., Ingalsbe, M. H., Benbow, J., & Daley, D. C. (2013). 12-Step interventions and mutual support programs for substance use disorders: An Overview. *Social Work in Public Health, 28*, 313–332.

Douaihy, A., & Daley, D. C. (Eds.). (2013). *Substance use disorders: Pittsburgh pocket psychiatry*. New York: Oxford University Press.

Douaihy, A. D., Kelly, T., & Gold, M. A. (Eds.). (2014). *Motivational interviewing: A guide for medical trainees*. New York: Guilford Press.

Fink, M. (1999). *Electroshock: Restoring the mind*. New York: Oxford University Press.

Fredrickson, B. L. (2009). *Positivity*. New York: Crown.

Galanter, M., & Kleber, H. D. (Eds.). (2015). *Textbook of substance abuse treatment*, 5th ed. Washington, DC: American Psychiatric Press.

Hester, R. K., & Miller, W. R. (Eds.). (2002). *Handbook of alcoholism treatment approaches: Effective alternatives*, 3rd ed. Boston: Allyn and Bacon.

Jansson, L. M., & Velez, M. L. (2010). Neonatal abstinence syndrome. *Current Opinion in Pediatrics, 24*(2), 252–258.

Kelly, J. F. (2016). *The science on the effectiveness and mechanisms of AA and 12-step treatments*. ATTC SAMHSA Webinar, April 21, 2016.

Kelly, J. F., Bergman, B., Hoeppner, B., Vilsaint, C., & White, W. L. (2017). Prevalence, pathways, and predictors of recovery from drug and alcohol problems in the United States population: Implications for practice, research, and policy. *Drug and Alcohol Dependence, 181*, 162–169.

Kelly, T. M., Daley, D. C., & Douaihy, A. B. (2012). Treatment of substance abusing patients with comorbid psychiatric disorders. *Addictive Behaviors, 37*(1), 11–24.

Kessler, R. C., Crum, R. M., Warner, L. A., Nelson, C. B., Schulenberg, J., & Anthony, J. C. (1997). Lifetime co-occurrence of DSM-III-R alcohol abuse and dependence with other psychiatric disorders in the national comorbidity survey. *Archives of General Psychiatry, 54*(4), 313–321.

Klostermann, K., & O'Farrell, T. J. (2013). Treating substance abuse: Partner and family approaches. *Social Work in Public Health, 28*(3-4), 234–247.

Kmiec, J., Cornelius, J., & Douaihy, A. (2013). Pharmacotherapy of substance use disorders. In A. Douaihy & D. Daley (Eds.), *Substance use disorders: Pittsburgh pocket psychiatry* (pp. 169–206). New York: Oxford University Press.

Laudet, A. (2013). *Life in recovery: Report on the survey findings.* Washington, DC: Faces and Voices of Recovery.

Marlatt, G. A., & Donovan, D. M. (Eds.). (2005). *Relapse prevention: Maintenance strategies in the treatment of addictive behavior,* 2nd ed. New York: Guilford Press.

McLellan, A. T., Lewis, D. C., O'Brien, C. P., & Kleber, H. D. (2000). Drug dependence, a chronic medical illness: Implications for treatment, insurance, and outcomes evaluation. *Journal of the American Medical Association, 284*(13), 1689–1695.

Miller, W. M., & Rollnick, S. (2013). *Motivational interviewing: Helping people change,* 3rd ed. New York: Guildford Press.

Monti, P., Adams, D., Kadded, R., Cooney, N., & Abrams, D. (2002). *Treating alcohol dependence,* 2nd ed. New York: Guilford Press.

Mueser, K., Noordsy, D. L., Drake, R. E., & Fox, L. (2003). *Integrated treatment for dual disorders: A guide to effective practice.* New York: Guilford Press.

Narcotics Anonymous World Services. (1988). *Narcotics Anonymous.* Van Nuys, CA: World Service Office, Inc.

Narcotics Anonymous World Services. (2015). *Narcotics Anonymous 2014 membership survey.* New York: Author.

National Institute on Alcohol and Alcoholism. (NIAAA). (2005). *Helping patients who drink too much: A clinician's guide.* Rockville, MD: USDHHS.

National Institute on Drug Abuse (1998). *Therapy manuals for drug addiction 1: A cognitive-behavioral approach to treating cocaine addiction.* Rockville, MD: Author.

National Institute on Drug Abuse. (1999). *Therapy manuals for drug addiction 3: An individual counseling approach to treat cocaine addiction.* Rockville, MD: Author.

National Institute on Drug Abuse. (2002). *Therapy manuals for drug addiction 4: Group drug counseling for cocaine addiction.* Rockville, MD: Author.

National Institute on Drug Abuse. (2012). *Principles of drug addiction treatment: A research-based guide,* 3rd ed. NIH Pub No. 12-4180. Rockville, MD: USDHHS.

Nowinski, J., & Baker, S. (1998). *The twelve-step facilitation handbook: A systematic approach to early recovery from alcoholism and addiction.* San Francisco: Jossey-Bass Publishers.

Onken, L. S., Blaine, J. D., & Boren, J. J. (1997). Treatment for drug addiction: It won't work if they don't receive it. *NIDA Research Monograph, 165,* 1–3.

Prochaska, J. O., DiClemente, C., & Norcross, J. C. (1992). In search of how people change: Applications to addictive behaviors. *American Psychologist, 47*(9), 1102–1114.

Project MATCH Research Group. (1998). Matching alcoholism treatment to client heterogeneity: Treatment main effects and matching effects on within treatment drinking. *Journal of Mental Health, 7*(6), 589–602.

Robins, L. N., & Regier, D. A. (1991). *Psychiatric disorders in America: The epidemiologic catchment area study.* New York: The Free Press.

Schukit, M. A. (2016). Treatment of opioid use disorders. *New England Journal of Medicine, 375,* 357–358.

Shea, S. C. (1999). *The practical art of suicide assessment: A guide for mental health professionals and substance abuse counselors.* New York: John Wiley & Sons.

Smith, E., & Daley, D. C. (2017). Substance use disorders and the family. In *Encyclopedia of abnormal and clinical psychology* (pp. 3378–3382). New York: SAGE Publications.

Smith, J. E., & Meyers, R. J. (2004). *Motivating substance abusers to enter treatment: Working with family members*. New York: Guilford Press.

Soyka, M. (2017). Treatment of benzodiazepine dependence. *New England Journal of Medicine, 376*(12), 1147–1157.

Substance Abuse and Mental Health Services Administration. (2015). *Medication for the treatment of alcohol use disorders: A brief guide*. HSS Publication No. (SMA) 15-4907. Rockville, MD: US Department of Health and Human Services.

Substance Abuse and Mental Health Services Administration. (2015). *Medication-assisted treatment of opioid use disorder*. HSS Publication No. (SMA) 14-4892R. Rockville, MD: US Department of Health and Human Services.

Substance Abuse and Mental Health Services Administration. (2016). *Building systems together for family recovery, safety and stability*. Webinar sponsored by SAMHSA and the Administration for Children and Families Children's Bureau.

Substance Abuse and Mental Health Services Administration. (2017). *2016 national survey on drug use and health*. Rockville, MD: SAMHSA.

Tarter, R. E., Kirisci, L., Mezzich, A., Cornelius, J. R., Pajer, K., Vanyu, M., et al. (2003). Neurobehavioral disinhibition in childhood predicts early stage at onset of substance use disorder. *American Journal of Psychiatry, 160*(6), 1078–1085.

Volkow, N. D., et al. (2014). Adverse health effects of marijuana use. *New England Journal of Medicine, 23*, 2219–2227.

White, W., & Daley, D. C. (2016). *Calling attention to opioid-affected families and children*. William L. White Blog, July 13, 2016. www.williamwhitepapers.com.

White, W. L. (2012). *Recovery/remission from substance use disorders: An analysis of reported outcomes in 415 scientific studies, 1868–2011*. Chicago: Great Lakes Addiction Technology Transfer Center; Philadelphia: Department of Behavioral Health and Developmental Disabilities; Pittsburgh, PA: Northeast Addiction Technology Transfer Center.

White, W. L. (2017). *Groundbreaking survey of recovery pathways*. November 3, 2017. www.williamwhitepapers.

White, W. L. (2017). *Recovery rising: A retrospective of addiction treatment and recovery advocacy*. Create Space Independent Publishing Platform.

**Dennis C. Daley, PhD,** is Senior Clinical Director of Substance Use Services in the Behavioral Health Integration Division at the UPMC Insurance Division. He is also a Professor of Psychiatry at the University of Pittsburgh School of Medicine. Dr. Daley has been involved in clinical care, research, and teaching about addiction for nearly 40 years. He has conducted hundreds of presentations in the United States, Canada, Europe, Mexico, Taiwan, and Vietnam.

Dr. Daley previously served for 14 years as Chief of Addiction Medicine Services at Western Psychiatric Institute and Clinic (WPIC) and for 11 years as the Director and Principal Investigator of the Appalachian Tri-State (ATS) Node of the National Institute on Drug Abuse's (NIDA) Clinical Trials Network, housed at WPIC. He has been an investigator, consultant, and trainer on numerous local and national studies.

He published the first book in the United States for counselors and the first recovery workbooks for individuals and families for substance use disorders and co-occurring psychiatric disorders. He was also one of the first in the United States to publish interactive workbooks on recovery from addiction. For decades, Dr. Daley has advocated for recovery for individuals and families affected by addiction.

Dr. Daley served on the Veteran Administration's MIRECC Project for more than 12 years in consulting and educational capacities related to addiction and mental health services for veterans. He has been involved in several national and local organizations that address substance use issues.

Dr. Daley has more than 400 publications, which include books, chapters, articles, and recovery guides. He writes regular columns for *Counselor* and other publications. He created more than 35 educational videos on recovery from addiction, mental health disorders, or co-occurring disorders, including the *Living Sober* series for addiction and the *Promise of Recovery* series for mental health disorders. His treatment manuals and his patient or family recovery materials are used in many programs in the United States and other countries. Several of his writings have been translated to foreign languages. He has also published material for children on under-standing substance use problems.

**Antoine Douaihy, MD,** is Professor of Psychiatry and Medicine at the University of Pittsburgh School of Medicine. He also serves as the senior academic director of Addiction Medicine Services and director of the Addiction Psychiatry Fellowship at Western Psychiatric Hospital of the University of Pittsburgh Medical Center. He has a well-established career in patient care/advocacy, education, training, and research in the areas of motivational interviewing, substance use disorders, co-occurring disorders, and HIV/AIDS. He and Dr. Daley have worked together for 20 years providing clinical services, conducting clinical research, teaching and mentoring healthcare practitioners and medical trainees, and publishing. In recognition of his dedication to an academic career, Dr. Douaihy has been the recipient of multiple awards, including the Leonard Tow Humanism in Medicine Award and the Charles Watson Teaching Award, recognizing him for the qualities of a masterful clinician, academician, caretaker of his patients, educator, mentor, and contributor to the medical school community and community at large.